S0-DPE-012

A Profile of
Health and Disease
in America

Mental
Illness and
Substance
Abuse

A Profile of
Health and Disease
in America

Mental Illness and Substance Abuse

Wrynn Smith, Ph.D.

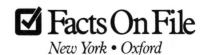

Facts On File
New York • Oxford

A Profile of Health and Disease in America:
Mental Illness and Substance Abuse

copyright © 1989 by Wrynn Smith

All rights reserved. No part of this book may
be reproduced or utilized in any form or by any
means, electronic or mechanical, including
photocopying, recording, or by any information
storage and retrieval systems, without permission
in writing from the publisher.

Library of Congress Cataloging-in-Publication Data

Smith, Wrynn.
  A profile of health and disease in America : mental illness and
substance abuse / Wrynn Smith.
       p.   cm.
  Bibliography: p.
  Includes index.

  1. Mental illness—United States—Statistics.   2. Substance abuse—
United States—Statistics.   3. Psychiatric epidemiology—United
States—Statistics.   4. United States—Statistics, Medical.
I. Title.
RC443.S58 1988
362.2′0973′021—dc19
  ISBN 0-8160-1457-4
  ISBN 0-8160-1588-0 (7 volume set)

Series design: Jo Stein

British CIP data available on request

Printed in the United States of America

10 9 8 7 6 5 4 3 2 1

CONTENTS

Preface

Just a few decades ago, treating the sick was a simple affair. The local family doctor, equipped with a small array of poultices and a sympathetic manner, did his best to fight disease. Knowledge, medicines, instrumentation, and surgical procedures developed slowly. Today, however, in the era of proliferating biotechnology, specialization, third-party financing, hospices, and surgicenters, medical school professors seem to relish telling their students that 50% of what they are learning will be obsolete five years after graduation.

The flow of information crossing the desk of busy health-care professionals trying to keep abreast of ever-accelerating developments in disease diagnosis, treatment, and prevention, as well as in the financing, organization, and delivery of health care, is often overwhelming. Clearly, the need to keep up is critical. To be informed, health-care professionals—be they practitioners, hospital administrators, health-care planners, policy makers, insurers, or hospital or pharmaceutical supply executives—must attend to material from many disconnected sources. These sources might include current editions of classic texts, weekly and monthly professional journals, current research papers presented at colloquia, and a steady stream of government bulletins and study publications from the Centers for Disease Control, NIH, the Center for Health Statistics, and foundation reports. As with the proverbial forest that can't be seen for the trees, the voluminous and fragmented form of this information often obscures the major changes and trends rapidly occurring in the health-care field.

The task of a grant applicant to locate and collate statistical information when framing the need for his work is a research project in itself. The same is true of a researcher defining a hypothesis, a physician determining the current utilization of a particular therapy regimen, or a hospital administrator projecting bed needs.

To help such workers and investigators, I decided to gather data from many sources into one comprehensive coordinated source, this series entitled *A Profile of Health and Disease in America*, that will serve as a handy and definitive resource tool for health professionals.

Each volume contains both historical and current statistics on the incidence, prevalence, and mortality of major diseases within one of the major medical specialties. I've presented data for different geographic areas within the United States as well as international data. I've also included information on the use of various medicines and surgical procedures. The length of a hospital stay, how it varies geographically or for patients based on sex, and treatment costs are included, as are discussions of major controversies. Thus, the reader will easily find data on flu viruses, changes in virus strains, current fertility rates of American teenagers, changes in the obesity level of Americans, and the latest incidence of pertussis, with a discussion of the pros and cons of the pertussis vaccine, and of how many men suffer from toxic shock syndrome. Those readers interested in digestive disease can find recent information from government surveys on problems as diverse as ulcers and hemorrhoids. The volume on mental disease provides a wealth of data on depressive symptomatology, drug usage, alcoholism, and homicide and puts the recent increase of teenage suicide in historical perspective.

Data sources include the 1983 Symposium on Cancer Treatment; Public Health Reports; the National Natality Survey; the NHANES Surveys; publications of the Atlanta Centers for Disease Control; and NIH publications, as well as those of the American Heart, Lung, and Blood Institute, The American Cancer Institute, and the Institute for Allergy and Infectious Disease. Published research articles are discussed and referenced, and each volume includes a bibliography that can be used by those seeking to go beyond initial review of pertinent health data. These comprehensive volumes on so many health topics need not be the last source consulted, but I think for those owning them they will always be the first.

Introduction

Mental disease seldom captures public or official attention or research dollars at any level that even approaches that directed toward purely physical diseases. Yet, as of 1980, a rough estimate of those persons receiving inpatient or outpatient treatment at public and private facilities was 3.25 million. This figure does *not* include the mentally retarded or another 1.4 million mental diagnosis discharges—including alcoholism—reported by general hospitals. Half of all hospital beds in the U.S. are occupied by the mentally ill. And it is estimated that about 1 of every 5 members of the general population suffer some form of mental illness.

The data described in this volume give a detailed picture of both the extent of major mental diseases and the resources devoted to treatment of the mentally ill. Inpatient and outpatient additions (repeat admissions within one year) at federally funded community mental health centers have increased, while they have decreased at state and county psychiatric facilities. Deinstitutionalization is reflected in the reduction of beds from 225.7 per 100,000 population (1972) to 123.2 (1980). Bed reductions at different types of facilities in each state are also noted, as is the change in the mix of facilities by type and the changed proportion of inpatient episodes from 77% of all treatment episodes in 1955 to 27% by 1977. During this time, total care episodes increased from 1.7 million to 6.9 million.

Occupancy rate and census counts also vary by facility and by state. Wyoming, e.g., has a low occupancy rate (13%) at community mental health centers, whereas the occupancy rate in Rhode Island's state and county mental health institutions is high (127%). Visits to physicians and psychiatrists according to mental diagnosis, treatment, and average duration of treatment provided are also reviewed. The supply of Ph.D. psychologists and residencies in psychiatry since 1960, the patients seen by different types of professionals, the work settings, and the full-time positions at various facilities are presented together with cost information. As of 1979, the per capita cost in state and county mental hospitals was $16.86 vs $6.65 at community mental health centers.

Chapter 2 presents survey information from the major epidemiologic catchment study conducted by the National Institutes of Mental Health (NIMH) of the noninstitutionalized population at several U.S. sites and from the federal government's Wellbeing Questionnaire survey of depression symptoms in the general population. The former study shows that 17% to 23% of the general population had a lifetime prevalence of at least one mental disorder. But only 23% of those persons who ever developed anxiety were treated, and only one-half of schizophrenics were ever treated. Age-related disorders, sex predominance, urban/rural residence, education level, and race correlates were also determined. The six-month prevalence of schizophrenia at 1.3% was slightly higher than the worldwide estimate of 1%.

Severe depression unrelated to bereavement was the most common disorder: 4 to 8 million depressed people were unable to function. According to the Wellbeing Questionnaire, 18.5 million persons reported symptoms, ranging from mild to severe, related to clinically pathologic or normal exogenous depression. Correlating race, sex, age, and economic variables were readily apparent. Those living in two- to four-person households excluding other variables were the least depressed.

Chapter 2 also furnishes extensive information on suicide in the United States and Europe. Roughly 26,000 people commit suicide in the U.S. each year: the rate has been fairly constant since 1960. However, the mix of those persons who commit suicide has changed markedly: there is a dramatic decrease among older people and an equally dramatic increase among younger ones. The same trend over several decades is seen in the European data.

Several hypotheses about the rise in suicide among young people are discussed. They include Durkheim's fragmentation theory (partly confirmed by trend predictions for European countries), changes in economic standing, pressure to achieve, reduced tolerance to stress, and the steady increase in the use of depression-causing drugs during the period in which the suicide rate rose. Often overlooked, drugs are a direct cause of suicidal depressions. The patterns of suicide in various countries for men and women, old and young, white and nonwhite are reviewed in detail, together with the success of suicide hotlines in England.

Information on other major forms of mental disease, such as neurosis, include data on the patients hospitalized, average length of stay, and prevalence in the general population. The 6-month prevalence of personality disorders for men is 2.1 vs 1.3 for women. The sociopathic or antisocial personality predominates in men.

Chapter 2 also supplies extensive information on the facilities for the residential mentally retarded by type of facility and state. It describes the educational programs for them under the Education for All Handicapped Children Act. At the other end of the age spectrum, organic brain damage is reviewed. Of persons older than age 80 years, 20% are thought to suffer from either Alzheimer's or senile dementia, a condition usually caused by vascular disease. Younger persons can also suffer organic brain damage caused by any of several diseases (head injury, alcoholism, or drug abuse), but the incidence is lower than in the elderly.

Alcohol and drug abuse can cause not only organic brain damage, but also acute depression and suicide; serious accidents; and psychoses, including schizophrenia, delusions, hallucinations, and violent criminal behavior. Persons suffering from mental disorders may also be more susceptible to substance abuse. Because of these relationships, alcohol and drug abuse are classified internationally with mental disorders.

Alcohol consumption in the United States has risen since the repeal of Prohibition. Currently 10 million people, or 7% of the population older than age 18 years, is thought to have a drinking problem. Indeed, 10% of all deaths are alcohol-related either as cirrhosis of the liver, accidents, suicide, homicide, or certain cancers. The chapter on alcohol abuse reviews the literature on the genetic cause of alcoholism; the MAST test and biologic markers used to diagnose it; and various treatments, including hospitalization, psychological support therapy, aversion therapy, and available treatment programs.

In 1982, there were 35,000 alcoholic patients in residential treatment programs; 202,917 received treatment at some kind of facility, including outpatient. Most of them, 116,198, were between age 21 and 44 years. The costs of alcohol treatment are carried by private health insurers (26%), government (10% local, 21% state), and several other sources.

Drug use and abuse have risen sharply in the United States since the early 1960s. An estimated 20 million people use marijuana, a usage that increased from 48% of the surveyed populations in 1972 to 68% in 1979. As of 1982, there was a slight decline among users age 12 to 17 years from 16.7% in the early 1970s to 11.5% in 1982. Cocaine is used regularly by 4 to 5 million Americans with no decline in sight as of the late 1980s. Information about violent antisocial behavior, personality disturbances, toxic psychoses with paranoid delusions and deep suicidal depressions, cardiac and respiratory deaths following use, especially IV use, has not yet spread to young adults. Their use jumped from 9.1% in 1972 to 28.5% in 1982. Almost 10% in this age group combined cocaine with marijuana.

Experimentation with heroin has been reported among ninth and tenth graders. Other opiates have been tried by students as early as the eighth grade. And 3.5% of high school seniors report they have used these drugs at least once. A steep decline in the use of hallucinogens, including LSD and PCP, was reported by high school graduating classes from 1980 through 1982: down from 14.5% in 1979 to 10.5% in 1982 as word spread about severe reactions, psychoses, and suicide following use of some of these substances.

Intravenous administration of amphetamines ("speed") can result in a personality modification that simulates schizophrenia more closely than any other drug sequela. Its use has also become more common; use of tranquilizers and barbiturates, however, has dropped since 1975, (although it rose slightly in the 1980s). Between 1975 and 1979, admissions to treatment for almost every popular illegal drug, except heroin, increased dramatically.

The causes of death, disease, and disability discussed in this volume illustrate the toll levied by genetic propensity and by voluntary individual behavior. Advances in genetic and biochemical research inspire hope that several of the mental diseases described may one day be known only in medical history. But the extent of death and illness that is self-inflicted supports either cynicism or optimism, depending on the resources and determination one believes society will ultimately expend to save people from themselves—a challenge greater than any science alone can meet.

Mental
Illness 1

Mental disease in one form or another has been observed
since earliest recorded history. In some societies, those
who heard voices and had hallucinations were regarded
as possessing special gifts. But in the West, the mentally ill have
often been regarded as possessed by evil spirits or punished by God
for wrongdoing. They have often been abused, persecuted, and even
killed. Flogging, starvation, and confinement in chains were common treatment for the insane during the Middle Ages.

PATIENT POPULATION

By the 18th and 19th centuries, medical practitioners were beginning to look more closely at the mentally ill. The leading hypothesis of the day was that some type of brain abnormality accounted for
mental disease. Today, the causes of mental disease are known to
be multiple; they comprise genetic, physical, social, environmental, and emotional factors.

The most serious mental disorders—schizophrenia, childhood
autism, and manic depression—are classified as psychoses. Less
severe are the many forms of neurosis: anxiety neurosis, neurotic
depression, hypochondria, phobia, hysteria, obsessive compulsive
neurosis, and depersonalization. Beyond these two categories of
illness are many personality or character disorders, or both.

Accurate assessment of persons with a mild or serious mental disease is difficult. One way to arrive at an estimate is by noting the patients who are outpatients or residents in public and private mental health treatment facilities at a given time, such as the end of a particular year. Table 1–1 shows the distribution of patients nationally and statewide for the end of various years in which recent data are available.

The total institutional resident patient year-end count in state and county facilities in 1980 plus those in private institutions at year's end 1979 was 146,471. General hospitals with psychiatric beds accounted for another 551,190 psychiatric discharge patients, not including 240,000 mentally retarded. Outpatient clinics reported 2,634,727 treatment episodes, including program admissions and readmissions.

If one adds the nearly 700,000 patients indicated in Table 1–1 (146,471 year-end inpatients plus the 551,471 general hospital psychiatric discharges) to the 2.7 million outpatient care episodes, the number of treated patients is roughly 3.25 million. But patient discharges and outpatient episodes do *not* accurately represent the number of persons treated. Patient discharges represent the number of treatment episodes; but, in one year, one patient may have several treatment episodes. Each succeeding episode after the first in a given year is an "addition." Thus, on the one hand, the estimate of 3.25 million mentally ill may be greatly inflated. On the other hand, many mentally ill people in the general population never enter the treatment system and the 3.25 million estimate may still be an underestimate of the true prevalence of mental illness.

ADDITIONS

Although additions are a misleading measure of the number of mentally ill, they can serve as an index of recidivism among patients treated. The readmission of an already-discharged patient may be inevitable. This is because the patient cannot always be relied on to continue his medication or his postdischarge follow-up therapy. Also, back-up community-based support services for a discharged patient or his family may be inadequate.

A large number of additions at an institution may also be a sign, however, of premature or inappropriate discharge policies. Since each repeat admission day requires a greater expenditure of resources than a typical care day during an ongoing program or stay in a facility, a high addition rate may signal an economically inefficient, indeed expensive, treatment policy. Extending the initial stay of a patient would be cheaper given this premise than releasing him sooner only to be readmitted again within months of his discharge.

Table 1–2 shows the inpatient additions for selected years between 1969 and 1979. The rate of readmission per 100,000 to public mental hospitals fell dramatically from 244.4 to 172.0, whereas the rate at private hospitals, V.A. psychiatric facilities, those for emotionally disturbed children, and federally funded community mental health centers rose.

Outpatient additions for selected years between 1969 and 1979 are shown in Table 1–3. Additions per 100,000 civilian population increased greatly between 1969 and 1979 at all facilities except state and county mental hospitals and private psychiatric hospitals.

Patients who are well enough to live in the community but who need more support than they can receive in a brief visit to an outpatient center often spend time at a day treatment center. The additions of day treatment center programs for selected years between 1969 and 1979 is shown in Table 1–4.

DEINSTITUTIONALIZATION

At one time, most people with mental disease were confined to residential facilities. As of the 1950s, however, several mind-controlling and mood-altering drugs were developed and used therapeutically for the mentally ill. In 1956, the number of resident patients in the United States fell for the first time in 175 years. This happened as patients whose symptoms were controlled by drugs were released for outpatient treatment. For years, authorities have estimated that one-half of the hospital beds in the United States are occupied by the mentally ill. Yet, the number of psychiatric beds has declined steeply in the 1970s from 225.7 per 100,000 population in 1972 to 123.2 in 1980 (Table 1–5).

Inpatient beds and the rate per 100,000 civilian population by type of facility in each state are shown in Table 1–6.

The decrease in psychiatric beds by state between 1972 and 1978 is shown in Figure 1–1. Ten states, (Maine, Vermont, New Hampshire, New Jersey, Indiana, Wisconsin, Minnesota, Nebraska, Nevada, and Alaska) decreased their bed count by 50% or more just in this 6-year period. Those states reducing beds the least were Utah, Colorado, Arizona, and New Mexico.

Interestingly, during the same 6 years, the homicide and suicide rates peaked and were particularly high in Nevada and Alaska. These concomitant developments may have been coincidental, but this observation speaks to one of the fiercest controversies surrounding the psychiatric-release policies of the last several years.

TABLE 1–1. Patients in Mental Health Facilities: 1977 to 1982 [Additions comprise admissions and readmissions]

REGION, DIVISION, AND STATE	MENTAL CARE HOSPITALS* — STATE AND COUNTY 1980 — Resident patients, end of year	MENTAL CARE HOSPITALS* — STATE AND COUNTY 1980 — Total additions	MENTAL CARE HOSPITALS* — PRIVATE 1979 — Resident patients, end of year	MENTAL CARE HOSPITALS* — PRIVATE 1979 — Total additions	OUTPATIENT PSYCHIATRIC SERVICES, ADDITIONS 1979*‡	GENERAL HOSPITALS WITH PSYCHIATRIC INPATIENT UNITS, DISCHARGES 1977*‡	STATE FACILITIES FOR MENTALLY RETARDED** — Resident patients 1982"	STATE FACILITIES FOR MENTALLY RETARDED** — Total admissions 1982	STATE FACILITIES FOR MENTALLY RETARDED** — Total live releases 1982	COMMUNITY FACILITIES, MENTALLY RETARDED RESIDENTS 1977¶‡
Facilities, number	280		185		2,431	843		245		4,427
United States	133,550	377,982	12,921	140,831	2,634,727	551,190	177,850	7,837	10,956	62,397
N. Eng.	7,777	30,173	1,753	14,497	209,968	19,877	8,993	1,807	467	3,930
Maine	654	1,335	—	—	16,292	438	403	285	267	629
N.H.	464	1,785	53	720	16,231	873	476	—	35	105
Vt.	256	620	62	651	8,981	397	280	5	26	220
Mass.	3,270	8,286	757	8,080	106,574	10,537	4,019	43	24	1,848
R.I.	723	4,173	145	2,323	16,124	1,067	561	7	115	182
Conn.	2,410	13,974	736	2,723	45,766	6,565	3,254	1,467	(NA)	947
Mid Atl.	41,421	50,304	2,113	22,781	478,651	98,065	25,695	1,018	3,123	10,205
N.Y.	25,530	33,766	637	5,318	286,397	59,921	12,768	(NA)	1,535	3,314
N.J.	5,468	8,958	404	3,752	62,626	13,552	6,280	864	1,052	789
Pa.	10,423	7,580	1,072	13,711	129,628	24,592	6,647	154	536	6,102
E. No. Cent.	18,144	61,711	1,736	20,318	454,289	113,906	17,471	959	1,908	15,250
Ohio	5,915	15,562	428	5,416	111,361	32,797	3,710	311	919	2,485
Ind.	2,769	6,599	—	—	82,552	12,959	2,810	95	176	479
Ill.	4,142	21,711	498	4,935	123,793	34,050	4,830	194	535	6,076
Mich.	4,464	13,750	576	7,929	92,969	18,527	3,967	247	179	4,126
Wis.	854	4,089	234	2,038	43,614	15,573	2,154	112	99	2,084
W. No. Cent.	9,524	42,294	315	1,917	196,581	59,200	8,481	589	754	9,424
Minn.	2,325	6,828	—	—	52,419	18,883	1,283	152	98	3,140
Iowa	1,097	6,086	—	—	24,822	11,682	1,684	83	136	1,150
Mo.	3,295	19,259	81	1,217	37,530	13,448	1,952	178	242	2,663
N. Dak.	570	2,538	—	—	11,609	1,969	1,000	9	36	185
S. Dak.	437	1,141	—	—	10,338	804	604	5	22	260
Nebr.	608	3,190	—	—	15,207	4,124	538	21	28	937
Kans.	1,192	3,252	234	700	44,656	8,290	1,420	141	192	1,089

So. Atl.	28,741	84,323	3,056	33,781	429,304	84,482	18,703	1,246	1,668	4,668
Del.	625	1,882	29	737	6,091	367	513	16	11	89
Md.	3,334	9,333	617	2,709	41,324	5,000	2,856	269	359	374
D.C.	2,088	4,949	143	1,545	16,672	4,022	950	–	6	40
Va.	4,839	10,099	739	8,492	48,777	13,172	3,471	170	211	508
W. Va.	1,746	1,863	46	1,310	23,267	5,400	481	49	38	56
N.C.	3,310	15,118	315	2,910	66,721	12,091	3,158	27	74	643
S.C.	3,233	6,526	–	–	30,784	5,333	3,000	178	181	310
Ga.	4,282	28,508	502	6,709	87,431	12,192	1,139	354	435	306
Fla.	5,284	6,045	665	9,369	108,237	26,905	3,135	183	353	2,342
E. So. Cent.	6,954	21,094	728	12,234	147,570	27,454	5,991	417	449	2,414
Ky.	554	2,406	357	5,741	47,486	7,500	677	20	13	950
Tenn.	2,614	10,189	166	2,178	43,575	8,558	2,172	100	86	903
Ala.	2,019	3,391	166	3,619	32,687	8,625	1,472	79	59	207
Miss.	1,767	5,108	39	696	23,822	2,771	1,670	218	291	354
W. So. Cent.	9,354	44,631	1,338	10,124	171,013	56,532	16,327	952	1,064	4,335
Ark.	256	2,062	–	–	32,875	2,677	1,365	26	77	215
La.	2,203	8,543	326	2,746	28,051	6,350	3,404	276	224	1,256
Okla.	1,190	8,376	40	723	34,529	6,673	1,803	118	128	584
Tex.	5,705	25,650	972	6,655	75,558	40,832	9,755	532	635	2,280
Mt.	2,945	11,413	359	5,003	173,389	19,344	4,273	285	452	2,644
Mont.	319	1,317	–	–	12,725	1,390	279	5	16	438
Idaho	213	523	–	–	11,054	990	351	15	19	266
Wyo.	261	749	–	–	12,291	–	441	7	34	101
Colo.	1,180	4,872	205	2,611	55,936	5,108	1,273	58	142	648
N. Mex.	227	1,702	57	793	16,428	755	503	46	35	206
Ariz.	324	697	97	1,599	39,682	5,786	525	25	83	343
Utah	306	640	–	–	14,403	3,376	742	37	41	412
Nev.	115	913	–	–	10,870	1,939	159	92	82	30
Pac.	8,690	32,039	1,523	20,176	373,962	72,330	11,916	564	1,071	9,527
Wash.	1,382	5,003	107	1,429	51,018	11,230	1,899	80	225	1,550
Oreg.	1,011	5,928	42	400	29,413	5,940	1,629	82	152	811
Calif.	5,915	19,262	1,374	18,347	280,710	53,875	7,921	376	653	6,870
Alaska	143	1,030	–	–	3,632	244	82	8	14	119
Hawaii	239	816	–	–	9,189	1,041	385	18	27	177

– Represents zero. NA not available. *Includes estimates for nonreporting facilities. †The latest data are shown for each facility type. Data for non-federal general and VA hospitals are for 1977; for federally funded community mental health centers, 1980, and for state and county mental hospitals, private psychiatric hospitals, freestanding psychiatric outpatient clinics and other facility types, 1979. ‡Non-federal. **Source: Rotegard and Bruininks Mentally Retarded People in State-Operated Residential Facilities: Years Ending June 30, 1981 and June 30, 1982, University of Minnesota, Minneapolis, Minn. Excludes facilities operated as mental hospitals or other care facilities. ¶As of June 30. "Admissions include readmissions. For year ending June 30.
Source: Statistical Abstracts of the United States, 1984

TABLE 1–2. Inpatient Additions, Percentage Distribution, and Rate per 100,000 Civilian Population, by Type of Mental Health Facility: United States, selected years 1969–79

TYPE OF FACILITY	1969	1971	1973	1975	1977	1979
	Inpatient additions					
All facilities	1,282,698	1,336,418	1,415,012	1,556,978	1,584,672	1,541,659
State and county mental hospitals	486,661	474,923	442,530	433,529	414,703	383,323
Private psychiatric hospitals	92,056	87,106	109,516	125,529	138,151	140,831
Nonfederal general hospital psychiatric services	478,000	519,926	468,415	543,731	551,190	551,190*
V.A. psychiatric services†	135,217	134,065	169,106	180,701	180,416	180,416*
Federally funded community mental health centers	59,730	75,900	183,026	236,226	257,347	246,409*
Residential treatment centers for emotionally disturbed children	7,596	11,148	12,179	12,022	15,152	15,453
All other facilities‡	23,438	33,350	30,240	25,240	27,713	24,037
	Percentage distribution of inpatient additions					
All facilities	100.0	100.0	100.0	100.0	100.0	100.0
State and county mental hospitals	37.9	35.6	31.3	27.8	26.2	24.9
Private psychiatric hospitals	7.2	6.5	7.7	8.1	8.7	9.1
Nonfederal general hospital psychiatric services	37.3	38.9	33.1	34.9	34.8	35.8*
V.A. psychiatric services†	10.5	10.0	12.0	11.6	11.4	11.7*
Federally funded community mental health centers	4.7	5.7	12.9	15.2	16.2	16.0*
Residential treatment centers for emotionally disturbed children	0.6	0.8	0.9	0.8	1.0	1.0
All other facilities‡	1.8	2.5	2.1	1.6	1.7	1.6
	Inpatient additions per 100,000 civilian population**					
All facilities	644.2	654.2	680.0	736.5	735.1	704.2
State and county mental hospitals	244.4	232.5	212.7	205.1	193.2	172.0
Private psychiatric hospitals	46.2	42.6	52.6	59.4	64.3	63.2
Nonfederal general hospital psychiatric services	240.1	254.5	225.1	257.2	256.7	256.7*
V.A. psychiatric services†	67.9	65.6	81.3	85.5	84.0	84.0*
Federally funded community mental health centers	30.0	37.2	88.0	111.7	119.9	110.6*
Residential treatment centers for emotionally disturbed children	3.8	5.5	5.8	5.7	7.1	6.9
All other facilities‡	11.8	16.3	14.5	11.9	12.9	10.8

Sources: *National Institute of Mental Health.* Statistical Note (SN) Series. Rockville, Md.: the Institute, and other published and unpublished sources, as follows: January 1971, 1975, 1977: SN 157, *Change in numbers of additions to mental health facilities, by modality, United States 1971, 1975, and 1977.* Sept. 1981. January 1969, 1973, 1979: National Institute of Mental Health. Unpublished data from the Division of Biometry and Epidemiology.

Notes: Information on facilities in Puerto Rico, Virgin Islands, Guam, and other U.S. territories are excluded. In tables where facilities and beds are shown, data are given at a point in time in January of a particular year.

*Since 1979 data are *not* available for V.A. psychiatric services, separate psychiatric services of nonfederal general hospitals, and federally funded community mental health centers (CMHCs); data are shown for 1980 for CMHCs and for 1977 for V.A. psychiatric services and separate psychiatric services of nonfederal general hospitals.

†Includes V.A. neuropsychiatric hospitals, V.A. general hospitals with separate psychiatric settings, and V.A. freestanding psychiatric outpatient clinics.

‡Includes other multiservice mental health facilities with an inpatient setting which are *not* elsewhere classified.

**The population used in the calculation of these rates is the civilian population of the United States for each year as provided by the Bureau of Census and published in Series P-25 publications.

TABLE 1–3. Outpatient Additions, Percentage Distribution, and Rate per 100,000 Civilian Population, by Type of Mental Health Facility: United States, selected years 1969–79

TYPE OF FACILITY	1969	1971	1973	1975	1977	1979
	Outpatient additions					
All facilities	1,146,612	1,378,822	1,714,030	2,289,779	2,343,360	2,634,727
State and county mental hospitals	164,232	129,133	167,647	146,078	107,692	81,919
Private psychiatric hospitals	25,540	18,250	31,656	32,879	33,573	30,004
Nonfederal general hospital psychiatric services	170,558	282,677	238,208	254,665	224,284	224,284*
V.A. psychiatric services†	16,790	51,645	68,016	93,935	120,243	120,243*
Federally funded community mental health centers	176,659	335,648	486,585	784,638	876,121	1,222,305*
Residential treatment centers for emotionally disturbed children	7,902	10,156	10,993	19,784	18,155	19,653
Freestanding psychiatric outpatient clinics	538,426	484,677	650,034	870,649	861,411	825,046
All other facilities‡	46,487	66,636	60,891	87,151	101,881	111,273
	Percentage distribution of outpatient additions					
All facilities	100.0	100.0	100.0	100.0	100.0	100.0
State and county mental hospitals	14.3	9.4	9.8	6.4	4.6	3.1
Private psychiatric hospitals	2.2	1.3	1.8	1.4	1.4	1.1
Nonfederal general hospital psychiatric services	14.9	20.5	13.9	11.1	9.6	8.5*
V.A. psychiatric services†	1.5	3.8	4.0	4.1	5.1	4.6*
Federally funded community mental health centers	15.4	24.3	28.4	34.3	37.4	46.5*
Residential treatment centers for emotionally disturbed children	0.7	0.7	0.6	0.9	0.8	0.7
Freestanding psychiatric outpatient clinics	47.0	35.2	37.9	38.0	36.8	31.3
All other facilities‡	4.0	4.8	3.6	3.8	4.3	4.2
	Outpatient additions per 100,000 civilian population**					
All facilities	575.9	674.9	823.7	1,083.2	1,091.5	1,188.4
State and county mental hospitals	82.5	63.2	80.6	69.1	50.2	36.8
Private psychiatric hospitals	12.8	8.9	15.2	15.6	15.6	13.5
Nonfederal general hospital psychiatric services	85.7	138.4	114.5	120.5	104.5	104.5*
V.A. psychiatric services†	8.4	25.3	32.7	44.4	56.0	56.0*
Federally funded community mental health centers	88.7	164.3	233.8	371.2	408.1	548.6*
Residential treatment centers for emotionally disturbed children	4.0	5.0	5.3	9.4	8.5	8.8
Freestanding psychiatric outpatient clinics	270.4	237.2	312.4	411.8	401.2	370.3
All other facilities‡	23.4	32.6	29.2	41.2	47.4	49.9

Sources: See Table 1–2.
Notes: Table 1–2.

*Since 1979 data are *not* available for V.A. psychiatric services, separate psychiatric services of nonfederal general hospitals, and federally funded community mental health centers (CMHCs); data are shown for 1980 for CMHCs and for 1977 for V.A. psychiatric services and separate psychiatric services of nonfederal general hospitals.
†Includes V.A. neuropsychiatric hospitals, V.A. general hospitals with separate psychiatric settings, and V.A. freestanding psychiatric outpatient clinics.
‡Includes freestanding psychiatric day/night facilities and other multiservice mental health facilities with an inpatient setting which are *not* elsewhere classified.
**The population used in the calculation of these rates is the civilian population of the United States for each year as provided by the Bureau of Census and published in Series P-25 publications.

TABLE 1–4. Day Treatment Additions, Percentage Distribution, and Rate per 100,000 Civilian Population, by Type of Mental Health Facility: United States, selected years 1969–79

TYPE OF FACILITY	1969	1971	1973	1975	1977	1979
			Day Treatment Additions			
All facilities	55,486	75,545	128,949	163,326	170,591	172,331
State and county mental hospitals	10,505	16,554	16,793	14,205	10,697	9,808
Private psychiatric hospitals	2,872	1,894	2,920	3,165	3,842	3,467
Nonfederal general hospital psychiatric services	18,094	11,563	18,772	14,216	12,724	12,724*
V.A. psychiatric services†	3,500	4,023	7,049	7,788	6,978	6,978*
Federally funded community mental health centers	13,011	21,092	59,130	94,092	102,493	98,332*
Residential treatment centers for emotionally disturbed children	671	994	1,666	3,431	3,147	2,519
Freestanding psychiatric outpatient clinics	4,387	10,642	15,329	21,928	21,149	29,587
All other facilities‡	2,446	8,783	7,300	4,501	9,561	8,916
			Percentage distribution of day treatment additions			
All facilities	100.0	100.0	100.0	100.0	100.0	100.0
State and county mental hospitals	18.9	21.9	13.0	8.7	6.3	5.7
Private psychiatric hospitals	5.2	2.5	2.3	1.9	2.3	2.0
Nonfederal general hospital psychiatric services	32.6	15.3	14.6	8.7	7.5	7.4*
V.A. psychiatric services†	6.3	5.3	5.5	4.8	4.1	4.0*
Federally funded community mental health centers	23.5	27.9	45.9	57.6	60.0	57.0*
Residential treatment centers for emotionally disturbed children	1.2	1.3	1.3	2.1	1.8	1.5
Freestanding psychiatric outpatient clinics	7.9	14.1	11.9	13.4	12.4	17.2
All other facilities‡	4.4	11.7	5.7	2.8	5.6	5.2

	Day treatment additions per 100,000 civilian population**					
All facilities	27.8	37.0	62.0	77.2	79.5	77.6
State and county mental hospitals	5.3	8.1	8.1	6.7	5.0	4.4
Private psychiatric hospitals	1.4	0.9	1.4	1.5	1.8	1.6
Nonfederal general hospital psychiatric services	9.1	5.7	9.0	6.7	5.9	5.9*
V.A. psychiatric services†	1.8	2.0	3.4	3.7	3.2	3.2*
Federally funded community mental health centers	6.5	10.3	28.4	44.5	47.7	44.1*
Residential treatment centers for emotionally disturbed children	0.3	0.5	0.8	1.6	1.5	1.1
Freestanding psychiatric outpatient clinics	2.2	5.2	7.4	10.4	9.9	13.3
All other facilities‡	1.2	4.3	3.5	2.1	4.5	4.0

Sources: See Table 1–2. Also:
1970: National Institute of Mental Health. Unpublished data from the Survey and Reports Branch, Division of Biometry and Epidemiology.
1972: *Utilization of Mental Health Facilities, 1971.* DHEW Pub. No. (NIH)74–657. Washington, D.C.: Supt. of Docs., U.S. Govt. Print. Off., 1973.
1974: SN 127, *Provisional data on patient care episodes in mental health facilities, 1973.* Feb. 1976.
1976: SN 139, *Provisional data on patient care episodes in mental health facilities, 1975.* August 1977.
1978: SN 154, *Trends in patient care episodes in mental health facilities, 1955–77.* Sept. 1980.
1980: National Institute of Mental Health. Unpublished data from the Survey and Reports Branch, Division of Biometry and Epidemiology.
Notes: See Table 1–2.

*Since January 1980 data are *not* available for V.A. psychiatric services, separate psychiatric services of nonfederal general hospitals, and federally funded community mental health centers (CMHCs); data are shown for February 1981 for CMHCs and for January 1978 for V.A. psychiatric services and separate psychiatric services of nonfederal general hospitals.
†Includes V.A. neuropsychiatric hospitals, V.A. general hospitals with separate psychiatric settings, and V.A. freestanding psychiatric outpatient clinics.
‡Includes freestanding psychiatric day/night facilities and other multiservice mental health facilities with an inpatient setting which are *not* elsewhere classified.
**The population used in the calculation of these rates is the civilian population of the United States for each year as provided by the Bureau of Census and published in Series P-25 publications.

TABLE 1–5. Bed and Bed Rates in Psychiatric Facilities, According to Type of Facility: United States, 1972, 1976, and 1980 (data are based on reporting by facilities)

TYPE OF FACILITY	Beds			Beds per 100,000 population		
	1972	1976	1980*	1972	1976	1980*
All facilities†	471,800	331,134	273,825	225.7	156.0	123.2
Nonfederal psychiatric hospitals	375,990	238,293	174,028	179.8	112.3	77.5
State and county hospitals	361,578	222,202	156,396	172.9	104.7	69.7
Private hospitals	14,412	16,091	17,632	6.9	7.6	7.8
Veterans Administration psychiatric services‡	42,545	35,913	33,796	20.3	16.9	15.7
Nonfederal general hospital psychiatric units	23,308	28,706	29,384	11.2	13.5	13.6
Residential treatment centers for emotionally disturbed children	19,348	18,029	20,197	9.3	8.5	9.0
Federally funded community mental health centers	10,609	10,193	16,420	5.1	4.8	7.4

Source: *National Institute of Mental Health*: State and regional distribution of psychiatric beds in 1972. *Statistical Note 98*. Public Health Service, Rockville, Md., Nov. 1973; State and regional distribution of psychiatric beds in 1976. *Statistical Note 144*. Public Health Service, Rockville, Md., Feb. 1978; State and regional distribution of psychiatric beds in 1978. *Statistical Note 155*. Public Health Service, Rockville, Md., Jan. 1981.

*Provisional data. 1980 data are not yet available for Veterans Administration neuropsychiatric hospitals, general hospital inpatient psychiatric units (Veterans Administration and nonfederal), and federally funded community mental health centers (CMHCs); 1979 data are used for CMHCs, and 1978 data are used for Veterans Administration psychiatric services and nonfederal general hospital psychiatric inpatient units.
†Excludes total inpatient days for multiservice mental health facilities not elsewhere classified which represent less than 1 percent of all inpatient days in each year.
‡Includes Veterans Administration neuropsychiatric hospitals and Veterans Administration general hospitals with separate psychiatric inpatient settings.

TABLE 1–6. Inpatient Beds and Rate per 100,000 Civilian Population, by Type of Mental Health Facility and State: United States, January 1980

STATE	All Facilities Number	Rate per 100,000 population¶	State and County Mental Hospitals Number	Rate per 100,000 population¶	Private Psychiatric Hospitals Number	Rate per 100,000 population¶	Nonfederal General Hospital Psychiatric Services* Number	Rate per 100,000 population¶	Federally Funded CMHCS† Number	Rate per 100,000 population¶	All Other Facilities‡*** Number	Rate per 100,000 population¶
Total, U.S.	274,713	124.3	156,482	70.2	17,157	7.7	29,384	13.7	16,264	7.3	55,426	25.4
Alabama	4,021	105.6	2,079	54.3	253	6.6	507	13.8	155	4.1	1,027	26.8
Alaska	145	38.0	133	34.9	–	–	12	3.1	–	–	–	–
Arizona	1,610	63.3	510	19.6	127	4.9	248	10.9	44	1.7	681	26.2
Arkansas	1,432	64.3	354	15.8	–	–	172	8.1	171	7.6	735	32.8
California	17,695	77.3	7,185	31.1	2,057	8.9	2,414	11.2	1,483	6.4	4,556	19.7
Colorado	3,269	117.0	1,180	42.0	305	10.8	221	8.6	155	5.5	1,408	50.1
Connecticut	4,855	156.8	2,443	79.0	816	26.3	393	12.7	124	4.0	1,079	34.8
Delaware	772	131.4	673	114.5	50	8.5	15	2.6	4	0.7	30	5.1
Dist. of Col.	2,818	440.3	2,171	340.8	199	31.2	185	27.1	13	2.0	250	39.2
Florida	9,937	107.8	6,196	66.2	966	10.3	1,285	15.4	568	6.1	922	9.8
Georgia	7,872	149.7	4,948	93.6	648	12.3	597	12.0	643	12.2	1,036	19.6
Hawaii	384	43.5	199	22.3	–	–	61	7.3	74	8.3	50	5.6
Idaho	430	46.7	266	28.7	–	–	28	3.3	14	1.5	122	13.2
Illinois	10,487	92.8	4,810	42.5	627	5.5	1,897	16.9	643	5.7	2,510	22.2
Indiana	6,569	120.8	3,596	65.9	–	–	759	14.3	807	14.8	1,407	25.8
Iowa	3,265	112.5	1,433	49.2	–	–	699	24.3	226	7.8	907	31.2
Kansas	3,208	137.5	1,343	57.4	273	11.7	495	21.5	304	13.0	793	33.9
Kentucky	2,668	74.9	958	26.7	471	13.1	376	11.0	296	8.3	567	15.8
Louisiana	3,580	87.6	2,512	61.1	486	11.8	346	8.9	72	1.8	164	4.0
Maine	1,604	145.2	690	62.4	–	–	22	2.0	66	6.0	826	74.8
Maryland	6,455	155.6	4,487	108.1	691	16.6	265	6.5	160	3.9	852	20.5
Massachusetts	9,946	173.3	3,489	60.8	859	15.0	688	11.9	1,002	17.5	3,908	68.1
Michigan	9,278	100.6	5,116	55.4	775	8.4	1,021	11.2	214	2.3	2,152	23.3
Minnesota	5,759	142.2	2,921	71.8	–	–	1,245	31.3	66	1.6	1,527	37.5
Mississippi	3,184	129.2	2,232	90.4	56	2.3	111	4.7	215	8.7	570	23.1
Missouri	6,033	124.0	3,527	72.3	100	2.0	856	17.9	696	14.3	854	17.5
Montana	702	89.6	469	59.7	–	–	56	7.4	81	10.3	96	12.2
Nebraska	1,299	83.4	827	53.0	–	–	235	15.2	109	7.0	128	8.2
Nevada	343	47.3	147	19.4	–	–	72	11.6	51	6.7	73	9.6
New Hampshire	788	87.2	494	54.5	56	6.2	31	3.7	71	7.8	136	15.0
New Jersey	9,882	134.8	6,900	94.1	460	6.3	828	11.3	389	5.3	1,305	17.8

continued

TABLE 1–6. Continued

				FACILITY							
STATE	All Facilities		State and County Mental Hospitals		Private Psychiatric Hospitals		Nonfederal General Hospital Psychiatric Services*		Federally Funded CMHCS†		All Other Facilities‡**	
	Number	Rate per 100,000 population¶	Number	Rate per 100,000 population¶	Number	Rate per 100,000 population¶	Number	Rate per 100,000 population¶	Number	Rate per 100,000 population¶	Number	Rate per 100,000 population¶
New Mexico	608	48.3	320	25.3	92	7.3	28	2.4	82	6.5	86	6.8
New York	39,292	223.4	27,647	157.4	870	5.0	3,243	18.1	854	4.9	6,678	38.0
North Carolina	38,260	145.8	4,148	72.9	431	7.6	612	11.3	1,865	32.8	1,204	21.2
North Dakota	909	141.3	788	122.4	–	–	102	15.9	19	3.0	–	–
Ohio	13,278	123.5	7,017	65.2	562	5.2	2,033	19.0	678	6.3	2,988	27.8
Oklahoma	3,223	109.8	2,469	83.6	93	3.1	378	13.6	93	3.1	190	6.4
Oregon	2,004	78.2	1,188	45.8	64	2.5	249	10.5	8	0.3	495	19.1
Pennsylvania	20,152	170.7	12,399	105.0	1,299	11.0	1,286	10.9	905	7.7	4,263	36.1
Rhode Island	1,140	121.7	736	78.6	168	17.9	48	5.2	35	3.7	153	16.3
South Carolina	4,269	143.1	3,614	120.7	–	–	262	9.3	245	8.2	148	4.9
South Dakota	1,097	160.3	548	80.1	–	–	54	7.9	176	25.7	319	46.6
Tennessee	5,453	121.8	3,165	70.3	275	6.1	507	11.9	329	7.3	1,177	26.2
Texas	13,217	97.1	6,911	50.1	1,291	9.4	2,116	16.7	283	2.0	2,616	18.9
Utah	892	64.2	367	25.8	–	–	170	13.5	85	6.0	270	18.9
Vermont	654	129.4	377	74.4	118	23.3	32	6.6	48	9.5	79	15.6
Virginia	8,481	165.0	5,629	109.3	1,125	21.8	609	12.2	194	3.8	924	17.9
Washington	2,677	67.7	1,347	33.6	131	3.3	354	9.8	113	2.8	732	18.2
West Virginia	2,862	149.0	2,154	111.8	54	2.8	227	12.2	304	15.8	123	6.4
Wisconsin	5,111	108.8	1,005	21.3	309	6.6	934	20.1	973	20.7	1,890	40.1
Wyoming	844	183.1	365	79.2	–	–			59	12.8	420	91.1

Source: *National Institute of Mental Health. Unpublished provisional estimates from the Survey and Reports Branch, Division of Biometry and Epidemiology.

Note: Information on facilities in Puerto Rico, Virgin Islands, and other U.S. territories are excluded.

*Since data for January 1980 are *not* available for nonfederal general hospital psychiatric inpatient services, data are shown for January 1978.

†Since data for January 1980 are *not* available for federally funded community mental health centers, data are shown for February 1981.

‡This category includes V.A. psychiatric services, residential treatment centers for emotionally disturbed children, and other multiservice inpatient mental health facilities which are *not* elsewhere classified.

**Since data for January 1980 are *not* available for V.A. psychiatric services, data are shown for January 1978.

¶The population used in the calculation of the rates is the civilian population by State as of January 1980, as provided by the Bureau of the Census.

Many opponents of patient-release policies question whether persons dangerous to themselves and/or others are being released into the general population. In the mid-1980s the general public and the media began taking more serious note of the growing number of homeless individuals inhabiting the nation's large cities. Both began to question the efficacy of returning many mentally ill people to the community without care, supervision, or protection.

FIG. 1–1.   Percentage change in the number of beds in all types of psychiatric facilities (excluding Community Mental Health Centers) per 100,000 population between 1972 and 1978, by state.

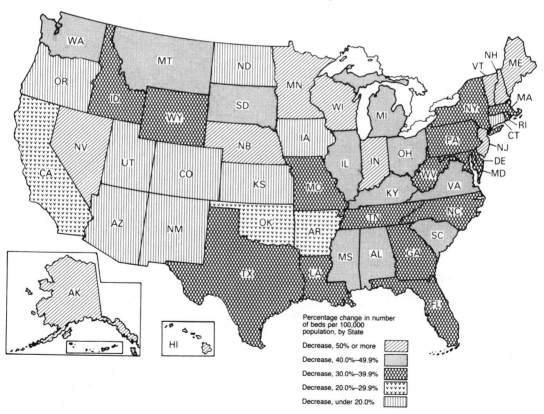

Source: *Mental Health Statistical Note* No. 155, DHHS, Jan. 1981

PATIENT CARE EPISODES

In 1955, 77% of all patient care was rendered in inpatient institutions. But by 1977, inpatient treatment accounted for only 27% of all patient-care episodes. The absolute number of care episodes in inpatient facilities in 1977 was about the same as in 1955, however, because patient-care episodes during this period rose fourfold, with a rapid rise in the patient turnover rate. (Figure 1–2).

The relative changes in patient treatment at different kinds of facilities is shown in Figure 1–3. Although inpatient treatment episodes have risen at some community mental health centers, most patient-care responsibility has been assumed by outpatient facilities. Increases shown in inpatient treatment facilities do not reflect a greater number of beds but rather a greater turnover of patients. Today, patients stay a shorter time in resident treatment than they once did.

TREATMENT FACILITIES

The shift away from residential treatment toward outpatient and day treatment has been accompanied by a change in the mix of facilities between 1970 and 1980 (Table 1–7). The federally funded community mental health center accounted for 6.5% of all mental health treatment facilities in 1970. But by 1980, these centers constituted 18.5% of all facilities.

The number of facilities by type in each state as of January 1980 is indicated in Table 1–8.

ADMISSIONS AND LENGTH OF STAY

The rate of admissions per 1,000 population at psychiatric bed facilities is shown in Table 1–9 for 1960 through 1981. Despite bed reductions, a faster patient turnover rate with many fewer days spent in the hospital during the 1970s compared to 1960 corresponded to an increasing admissions rate that did not taper off until the late seventies.

The trend in days of stay at different kinds of facilities since the 1970s is shown in Table 1–10. The total number of inpatient days per 1,000 population for all facilities has decreased markedly from 848.5 to 386.0. This reduction is mostly in state and county mental hospitals. The rates in general hospitals, federally funded community mental health centers and residential centers for the emotionally disturbed have all risen.

FIG. 1–2. Percentage distribution of patient care episodes in mental health facilities by modality: United States, 1955, 1971, 1975, 1977

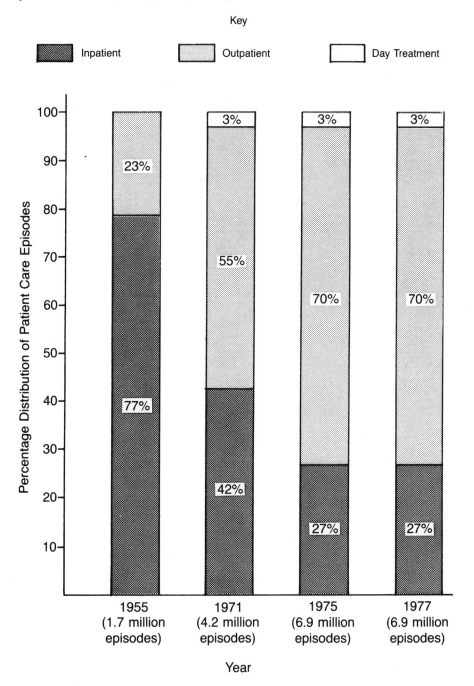

Source: *Mental Health Statistical Note* No. 154 DHHS September 1980

FIG. 1–3. Inpatient and outpatient care episodes per 100,000 population by type of facility and modality: United States, 1955, 1965, 1971, 1975, 1977

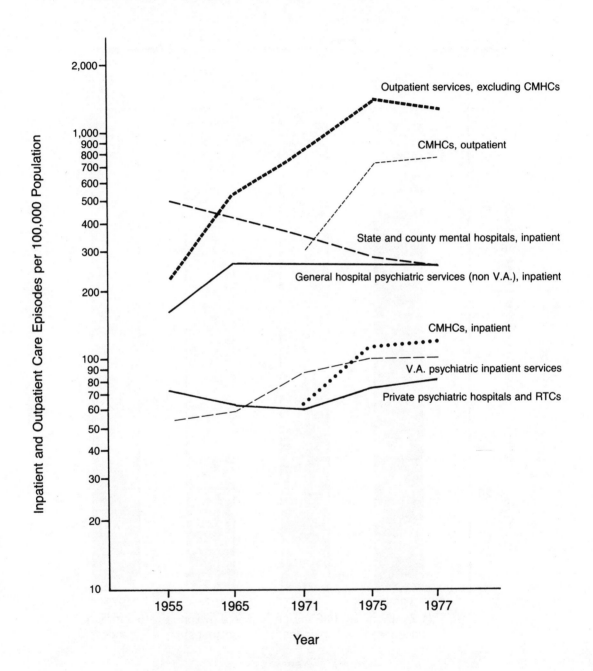

Source: *Mental Health Statistical Note* No. 154 DHHS September 1980
Key: CMHCs, community mental health centers; RTCs, residential treatment centers

TABLE 1–7. Number and Percentage Distribution of Mental Health Facilities, by Type of Facility: United States, selected years 1970–80

TYPE OF FACILITY	1970	1972	1974	1976	1978	1980
	Number of mental health facilities					
All facilities	3,005	3,187	3,315	3,480	3,738	3,727
State and county mental hospitals	310	321	320	303	297	280
Private psychiatric hospitals	150	156	180	182	188	184
Nonfederal general hospitals with separate psychiatric services	797	770	796	870	923	923*
V.A. psychiatric services†	115	119	119	126	136	136*
Federally funded community mental health centers	196	287	391	517	555	691*
Residential treatment centers for emotionally disturbed children	261	344	340	331	375	368
Freestanding psychiatric outpatient clinics	1,109	1,123	1,092	1,076	1,160	1,053
All other facilities‡	67	67	77	75	104	92
	Percentage distribution of mental health facilities					
All facilities	100.0	100.0	100.0	100.0	100.0	100.0
State and county mental hospitals	10.3	10.1	9.7	8.7	8.0	7.5
Private psychiatric hospitals	5.0	4.9	5.4	5.2	5.0	4.9
Nonfederal general hospitals with separate psychiatric services	26.5	24.2	24.0	25.0	24.7	24.8*
V.A. psychiatric services†	3.8	3.7	3.6	3.6	3.6	3.6*
Federally funded community mental health centers	6.5	9.0	11.8	14.9	14.9	18.5*
Residential treatment centers for emotionally disturbed children	8.7	10.8	10.3	9.5	10.0	9.9
Freestanding psychiatric outpatient clinics	36.9	35.2	32.9	30.9	31.0	28.3
All other facilities‡	2.3	2.1	2.3	2.2	2.8	2.5

Sources: *National Institute of Mental Health.* Statistical Note (SN) Series. Rockville, Md.: the Institute, and other published and unpublished sources, as follows: (1971, 1975, 1977). SN 157. *Changes in the numbers of additions to mental health facilities, by modality, United States, 1971, 1975, and 1977,* Sept. 1981. (1969, 1973, 1979): National Institute of Mental Health. Unpublished data from Survey and Reports Branch, Division of Biometry and Epidemiology.

Notes: See Table 1–2.

*Since 1979 data are *not* available for V.A. psychiatric services, separate psychiatric services of nonfederal general hospitals, and federally funded community mental health centers (CMHCs), data are shown for 1980 for CMHCs and for 1977 for V.A. psychiatric services and separate psychiatric services of nonfederal general hospitals.
†Includes V.A. neuropsychiatric hospitals, V.A. general hospitals with separate psychiatric settings, and V.A. freestanding psychiatric outpatient clinics.
‡Includes freestanding psychiatric day/night facilities and other multiservice mental health facilities with an inpatient setting which are *not* elsewhere classified.

TABLE 1–8. Mental Health Facilities, by Type of Facility and State: United States, January 1980

STATE	State and County Mental Hospitals	Private Psychiatric Hospitals	Nonfederal General Hospital Psychiatric Services*	V.A. Psychiatric Services†	Federally Funded CMHCs‡	RTCs for Emotionally Disturbed Children	Freestanding Psychiatric Outpatient Clinics	Freestanding Psychiatric Day/Night Facilities	All Other**
Total, U.S.	280	184	923	136	691	368	1,053	53	39
Alabama	4	3	15	3	20	2	6	–	–
Alaska	1	–	1	–	2	–	13	–	–
Arizona	1	2	8	2	7	9	10	–	2
Arkansas	1	–	5	1	14	2	3	1	–
California	6	28	79	10	45	39	68	7	18
Colorado	3	4	11	2	17	17	5	–	1
Connecticut	8	6	21	2	8	13	27	1	–
Delaware	2	1	1	1	2	–	3	–	1
Dist. of Col.	1	1	8	1	3	2	3	–	1
Florida	6	12	32	4	35	4	21	1	–
Georgia	8	8	19	2	25	4	12	1	–
Hawaii	1	–	8	–	6	1	4	–	–
Idaho	2	–	2	1	5	2	2	1	–
Illinois	15	5	48	5	20	16	79	9	2
Indiana	8	–	20	2	22	5	8	–	–
Iowa	5	–	19	3	6	4	28	–	–
Kansas	3	2	14	3	10	2	10	–	1
Kentucky	5	2	16	2	19	4	2	–	1
Louisiana	5	4	11	3	15	2	11	–	–
Maine	2	–	2	1	8	5	1	–	–
Maryland	6	6	14	2	10	7	34	3	–
Massachusetts	8	9	38	6	24	27	49	3	1
Michigan	12	8	35	3	20	21	59	–	–
Minnesota	6	–	26	2	5	12	22	–	–

State									
Mississippi	2	1	6	2	14	—	—	—	—
Missouri	8	1	23	4	13	12	20	—	—
Montana	1	—	3	—	5	1	—	—	—
Nebraska	4	—	4	2	7	1	4	—	—
Nevada	2	—	3	1	2	2	1	—	—
New Hampshire	1	1	3	1	7	3	3	—	—
New Jersey	10	3	28	2	22	8	32	6	—
New Mexico	1	1	2	1	5	1	10	—	—
New York	32	12	84	11	25	26	138	6	3
North Carolina	4	5	23	4	27	8	12	—	3
North Dakota	1	—	4	—	5	—	2	—	—
Ohio	18	7	56	5	28	21	72	2	—
Oklahoma	3	1	11	2	8	3	29	—	—
Oregon	2	1	9	2	2	6	27	1	1
Pennsylvania	18	13	57	6	41	6	69	6	—
Rhode Island	1	2	3	1	6	3	12	—	—
South Carolina	4	—	9	2	14	2	5	—	1
South Dakota	1	—	3	2	4	2	4	—	—
Tennessee	5	3	16	4	21	2	13	1	1
Texas	10	12	43	7	28	12	14	—	1
Utah	1	—	7	1	9	3	3	—	—
Vermont	1	1	1	1	6	5	1	—	—
Virginia	10	12	19	3	12	7	24	1	1
Washington	2	2	17	5	11	9	30	2	—
West Virginia	4	1	6	2	10	2	5	—	—
Wisconsin	14	4	30	3	7	21	38	2	—
Wyoming	1	—	—	1	4	2	5	—	—

Source: *National Institute of Mental Health.* Unpublished provisional estimates from the Survey and Reports Branch, Division of Biometry and Epidemiology.
Note: Information on facilities in Puerto Rico, Virgin Islands, and other U.S. territories are excluded.
*Since data for January 1980 are *not* available for nonfederal general hospital psychiatric inpatient services, data are shown for January 1978.
†Since data for January 1980 are *not* available for V.A. psychiatric services, data are shown for January 1978.
‡Since data for January 1980 are *not* available for federally funded community mental health centers, data are shown for February 1981.
***This category includes other multiservice mental health facilities with an inpatient setting which are *not* elsewhere classified.

TABLE 1–9. Trend in Hospital Psychiatric Admissions, 1960–1981

	19									
ADMISSIONS RATE PER 1,000 POPULATION	'60	'65	'70	'75	'76	'77	'78	'79	'80	'81
	2.3	2.9	3.3	3.2	3.1	3.0	2.9	2.8	2.8	2.7

The total number of inpatient days in thousands and the rate per 1,000 civilian population by type of facility in each state for 1979 are indicated in Table 1–11.

Data on discharges and average length of stay in days for mental patients by diagnosis and sex are presented in Table 1–1. Women have a longer average length of stay than men for most diagnoses.

Table 1–13 presents data on the length of stay for patients with various diagnoses according to their age. The youngest and oldest patients have the longest length of stay for several diagnostic categories.

PATIENT CENSUS

The patient census is a valuable measure of utilization. The occupancy rate in various states varies from 68.8% for all facilities in Montana and Wyoming to 127% in Rhode Island in state and county mental hospitals (Table 1–14). In federally funded CMHCs (community mental health centers) the occupancy rates varied from only 13.6% in Wyoming to 121% in North Dakota.

The inpatient census for the United States from 1969 to 1979 in different types of facilities is shown in Table 1–15. The daily census for all facilities during this period dropped by almost 50%. Not every type of facility, however, showed this decline.

MENTAL HEALTH TREATMENT AND RESOURCES

In 1980, there were 24,343 visits to physicians by people whose principal diagnosis was a mental disorder (Table 1–16). Another 32,518 visits were made by people with a diagnosis of mental disturbance in addition to their principal diagnosis.

Among patients with a mental disorder as their principal diagnosis, neurosis and affective (depression) disorders accounted for most visits made to psychiatrists and to physicians in all specialties.

TABLE 1–10. Inpatient Days in Thousands, Percent Distribution, and Rate per 1,000 Civilian Population, by Type of Mental Health Facility: United States, selected years 1969–79

TYPE OF FACILITY	1969	1971	1973	1975	1977	1979
	Number of inpatient days in thousands					
All facilities	168,934	153,639	126,375	104,970	92,084	85,285
State and county mental hospitals	134,185	119,200	92,210	70,584	57,206	50,589
Private psychiatric hospitals	4,237	4,220	4,108	4,401	4,792	5,074
Nonfederal general hospital psychiatric services	6,500	6,826	6,990	8,349	8,435	8,435*
V.A. psychiatric services†	17,206	14,277	12,985	11,725	10,628	10,628*
Federally funded community mental health centers	1,924	2,225	3,276	3,718	3,818	3,609*
Residential treatment centers for emotionally disturbed children	4,528	6,356	6,338	5,900	6,546	6,531
All other facilities‡	354	535	468	293	659	419
	Distribution of inpatient days (%)					
All facilities	100.0	100.0	100.0	100.0	100.0	100.0
State and county mental hospitals	79.4	77.6	73.0	67.2	62.1	59.3
Private psychiatric hospitals	2.5	2.8	3.2	4.2	5.2	5.9
Nonfederal general hospital psychiatric services	3.9	4.4	5.5	8.0	9.2	9.9*
V.A. psychiatric services†	10.2	9.3	10.3	11.2	11.5	12.5*
Federally funded community mental health centers	1.1	1.5	2.6	3.5	4.2	4.2*
Residential treatment centers for emotionally disturbed children	2.7	4.1	5.0	5.6	7.1	7.7
All other facilities‡	0.2	0.3	0.4	0.3	0.7	0.5
	Inpatient days per 1,000 civilian population**					
All facilities	848.5	752.1	607.2	496.6	428.9	386.0
State and county mental hospitals	674.0	583.5	443.1	333.9	266.4	227.1
Private psychiatric hospitals	21.3	20.7	19.7	20.8	22.3	22.8
Nonfederal general hospital psychiatric services	32.6	33.4	33.6	39.5	39.3	39.3*
V.A. psychiatric services†	86.4	69.9	62.4	55.5	49.5	49.5*
Federally funded community mental health centers	9.7	10.9	15.7	17.6	17.8	16.2*
Residential treatment centers for emotionally disturbed children	22.7	31.1	30.5	27.9	30.5	29.3
All other facilities‡	1.8	2.6	2.2	1.4	3.1	1.8

Source (1969, 1979): *National Institute of Mental Health*. Unpublished data from the Survey and Reports Branch, Division of Biometry and Epidemiology; (1971, 1973, 1975, 1977): Regier, D.A., and Taube, C.A. The delivery of mental health services. In *American Handbook of Psychiatry*, 7. New York: Basic Books, 1981.
Notes: Information on facilities in Puerto Rico, Virgin Islands, Guam, and other U.S. Territories are excluded. In tables where facilities and beds are shown, data are given at a point in time in January of a particular year.
*Since 1979 data are *not* available for V.A. psychiatric services, separate psychiatric services of nonfederal general hospitals, and federally funded community mental health centers (CMHCs), data are shown for 1980 for CMHCs and for 1977 for V.A. psychiatric services and separate psychiatric services of nonfederal general hospitals.
†Includes V.A. neuropsychiatric hospitals, V.A. general hospitals with separate psychiatric settings, and V.A. freestanding psychiatric outpatient clinics.
‡Includes other multiservice mental health facilities with an inpatient setting which are *not* elsewhere classified.
**The population used in the calculation of these rates is the civilian population of the United States for each year as provided by the Bureau of the Census and published in Series P-25 publications.

TABLE 1–11. Inpatient Days in Thousands and Rate per 1,000 Civilian Population, by Type of Mental Health Facility and State: United States, 1979

| STATE | All Facilities | | TYPE OF FACILITY | | | | | | | | | |
| | | | State and County Mental Hospitals | | Private Psychiatric Hospitals | | Nonfederal General Hospital Psychiatric Services* | | Federally Funded CMHCs† | | All Other Facilities†** | |
	Number in 000s	Rate per 1,000 population¶	Number in 000s	Rate per 1,000 population¶	Number in 000s	Rate per 1,000 population¶	Number in 000s	Rate per 1,000 population¶	Number in 000s	Rate per 1,000 population¶	Number in 000s	Rate per 1,000 population¶
Total, U.S.	85,285	386.0	50,589	227.1	5,074	22.8	8,435	39.3	3,609	16.2	17,578	80.7
Alabama	1,215	318.7	726	189.7	55	14.4	109	29.7	25	6.5	300	78.4
Alaska	51	133.8	50	131.2	—	—	1	2.6	—	—	—	—
Arizona	518	203.4	183	70.3	35	13.4	80	35.2	11	4.2	209	80.3
Arkansas	388	174.4	83	37.1	—	—	51	23.9	34	15.2	220	98.2
California	5,286	231.0	2,296	99.5	579	25.1	671	31.0	419	18.2	1,321	57.2
Colorado	1,006	359.8	352	125.2	90	32.0	61	23.7	40	14.2	463	164.7
Connecticut	1,590	513.4	801	258.6	277	89.4	132	42.7	53	17.1	327	105.6
Delaware	252	428.7	223	379.3	16	27.2	4	6.9	1	1.7	8	13.6
Dist. of Col.	910	1,422.9	718	1,127.2	61	95.8	55	80.6	3	4.7	73	114.6
Florida	3,175	343.6	2,101	224.4	256	27.3	350	41.9	140	15.0	328	35.0
Georgia	2,263	429.8	1,570	297.1	201	38.0	136	27.3	124	23.5	232	43.9
Hawaii	101	114.1	55	61.7	—	—	12	14.3	18	20.2	16	17.9
Idaho	112	121.9	74	79.9	—	—	9	10.6	2	2.2	27	29.2
Illinois	3,423	305.1	1,504	132.9	190	16.8	707	63.1	179	15.8	843	74.5
Indiana	1,936	356.1	1,099	201.5	—	—	246	46.2	163	29.9	428	78.5
Iowa	945	325.6	417	143.3	—	—	202	70.2	38	13.1	288	99.0
Kansas	959	410.6	402	171.7	90	38.4	122	53.1	88	37.6	257	109.8
Kentucky	743	208.7	296	82.6	101	28.2	104	30.4	46	12.8	196	54.7
Louisiana	1,148	280.4	851	206.9	144	35.0	95	24.4	15	3.6	43	10.5
Maine	531	480.7	219	198.2	—	—	6	5.6	18	16.3	288	260.6
Maryland	1,968	474.0	1,369	329.7	238	57.3	36	8.8	45	10.8	280	67.4
Massachusetts	3,125	544.5	1,051	183.2	282	49.2	224	38.8	268	46.7	1,300	226.6

State										
Michigan	2,926	317.3	178.7	248	26.9	312	34.2	50	5.4	666	72.1
Minnesota	1,736	428.8	213.5	—	—	375	94.4	15	3.7	477	117.2
Mississippi	951	385.6	283.4	21	8.5	33	13.9	22	8.9	175	70.9
Missouri	1,787	367.3	228.8	34	7.0	265	55.5	122	25.0	249	51.0
Montana	174	221.8	173.2	—	—	4	5.3	5	6.4	29	36.9
Nebraska	369	236.9	157.1	—	—	63	40.7	19	12.2	42	26.9
Nevada	102	139.6	63.4	—	—	17	27.3	12	15.9	25	33.0
New Hampshire	280	309.5	208.4	20	22.1	9	10.7	14	15.4	48	52.9
New Jersey	3,022	412.3	309.1	160	21.8	124	17.0	110	15.0	362	49.4
New Mexico	196	155.4	93.3	20	15.8	8	6.8	21	16.6	29	22.9
New York	13,612	773.9	558.2	252	14.3	1,064	59.4	270	15.4	2,223	126.6
North Carolina	2,318	408.9	224.8	106	18.6	182	33.5	236	41.5	515	90.5
North Dakota	262	407.1	344.7	—	—	31	48.4	9	14.0	—	—
Ohio	3,886	361.5	198.6	168	15.6	648	60.6	156	14.5	777	72.2
Oklahoma	909	310.3	237.4	18	6.1	112	40.3	22	7.5	56	19.0
Oregon	600	233.6	139.5	15	5.8	67	28.2	2	0.8	154	59.3
Pennsylvania	6,221	526.8	315.3	412	34.9	338	28.7	272	23.0	1,475	124.9
Rhode Island	474	506.6	366.5	53	56.6	17	18.3	9	9.6	52	55.6
South Carolina	1,392	466.1	406.3	—	—	63	22.4	66	22.0	46	15.4
South Dakota	310	453.3	260.2	—	—	12	17.6	14	20.5	106	155.0
Tennessee	1,738	387.8	240.9	70	15.6	137	32.0	59	13.1	388	86.2
Texas	3,883	284.7	148.7	388	28.1	527	41.6	61	4.4	854	61.9
Utah	223	158.8	82.8	—	—	26	20.6	19	13.3	60	42.1
Vermont	223	440.8	260.4	45	88.8	9	18.6	11	21.7	26	51.3
Virginia	2,633	512.3	367.8	283	55.0	152	30.5	50	9.7	254	49.3
Washington	871	219.6	112.7	33	8.2	89	24.7	23	5.7	274	68.3
West Virginia	882	446.1	371.8	18	9.3	73	39.3	43	9.1	32	16.6
Wisconsin	1,447	307.9	65.4	95	20.2	265	57.0	164	34.8	615	130.5
Wyoming	213	462.0	190.9	—	—	—	—	3	6.5	122	264.4

Source: *National Institute of Mental Health.* Unpublished provisional estimates from the Survey and Reports Branch, Division of Biometry and Epidemiology.

Note: Information on facilities in Puerto Rico, Virgin Islands, and other U.S. territories are excluded.

*Since data for 1979 are *not* available for nonfederal general hospital psychiatric inpatient services, data are shown for 1977.

†Since data for 1979 are *not* available for federally funded community mental health centers, data are shown for 1980.

‡This category includes V.A. psychiatric services, residential treatment centers for emotionally disturbed children, and other multiservice mental health facilities with an inpatient setting which are *not* elsewhere classified.

**Since data for 1979 are *not* available for V.A. psychiatric services, data are shown for 1977.

¶The population used in the calculation of the rates is the civilian population by State as of January 1980, as provided by the Bureau of the Census.

TABLE 1–12. Number and Percentage Distribution of Mental Disorder Discharges from Nonfederal Short-stay Hospitals, by Sex and Average Length of Stay: United States, 1980

FIRST-LISTED DIAGNOSIS	DISCHARGES						AVERAGE LENGTH OF STAY IN DAYS		
	Total		Male		Female		Total	Male	Female
	Number (in 000s)	Percent	Number (in 000s)	Percent	Number (in 000s)	Percent			
All first-listed diagnoses	1,692	100.0	855	100.0	807	100.0	11.6	10.9	12.2
Mental retardation	12	0.7	5	0.6	7	0.9	11.2	7.5	13.9
Alcohol and drug related disorders	602	35.6	455	51.5	147	18.2	9.6	9.5	9.8
Organic brain syndromes other than alcohol and drug related	124	7.3	55	6.2	69	8.5	13.4	12.9	13.7
Affective disorders	325	19.2	103	11.6	222	27.5	14.1	13.1	14.6
Schizophrenia and related disorders	183	10.8	96	10.9	86	10.7	16.1	15.7	16.7
Other psychoses	53	3.1	24	2.8	28	3.5	13.0	11.2	14.6
Neuroses other than depressive	133	7.8	46	5.1	87	10.8	6.2	6.4	6.0
Personality disorders	54	3.2	25	2.8	29	3.6	13.5	11.7	15.1
Pre-adult disorders	10	0.6	7	0.8	*	*	18.5	21.3	*
Other mental disorders	197	11.7	68	7.7	129	16.0	10.2	10.6	10.0

Source: *National Institute of Mental Health.* Compiled from unpublished data from the National Hospital Discharge Survey.

TABLE 1–13. Average Length of Stay of Mental Disorder Discharges from Nonfederal Short-stay Hospitals, by First-listed Diagnosis and Age: United States, 1980

| FIRST-LISTED DIAGNOSIS | Total | LENGTH OF STAY IN DAYS BY AGE | | | |
		Under 15 years	15 to 44 years	45 to 64 years	65 years and over
All first-listed diagnoses	11.5	13.5	11.0	11.3	13.7
Mental retardation	11.2	–	11.6	–	–
Alcohol and drug related disorders	9.6	6.5	9.5	9.9	9.5
Organic brain syndromes other than alcohol and drug related	13.4	–	10.0	10.9	14.9
Affective disorders	14.1	–	12.0	15.5	18.0
Schizophrenia and related disorders	16.1	–	16.1	15.1	17.9
Other psychoses	13.0	–	11.9	15.1	13.4
Neuroses other than depressive	6.2	4.2	6.2	6.6	6.0
Personality disorders	13.5	–	12.8	12.7	–
Pre-adult disorders	18.5	17.0	–	–	–
Other mental disorders	10.2	13.1	10.1	9.1	11.5

Source: *National Institute of Mental Health.* Compiled from unpublished data from the National Hospital Discharge Survey.

TABLE 1–16. Percentage Distribution of Office Visits to All Physicians in Which There Was a Principal or Any Diagnosis of Mental Disorder, by Patient, Sex, Color, and Age: United States, 1980

| SEX, COLOR, AND AGE | ALL VISITS | VISITS WITH A DIAGNOSIS OF MENTAL DISORDER | |
		Principal diagnosis	Any diagnosis
Number of visits (in 000s)	575,745	24,343	32,518
Percent	100.0	100.0	100.0
Sex:			
Male	39.9	39.3	37.7
Female	60.1	60.7	62.3
Color:			
White	89.7	92.4	92.1
All other	10.3	7.6	7.9
Age (years):			
0–17	22.4	5.1	5.8
18–24	10.7	7.7	6.7
25–44	26.9	51.4	44.8
45–64	22.6	26.4	29.7
65+	17.4	9.3	13.0

Source: *National Institute of Mental Health.* Compiled from unpublished data from the National Ambulatory Medical Care Survey.

TABLE 1–14. Average Daily Inpatient Census and Percentage Occupancy, by Type of Mental Health Facility and State: United States, 1979

STATE	All facilities		State and county mental hospitals		Private psychiatric hospitals		Nonfederal general hospital psychiatric services*		Federally funded CMHCs†		All other facilities‡**	
	Average daily census	Percent occupancy	Average daily census	Percent occupancy	Average daily census	Percent occupancy	Average daily census	Percent occupancy	Average daily census	Percent occupancy	Average daily census	Percent occupancy
Total, U.S.	233,384	85.0	138,600	88.6	13,901	81.0	23,110	78.6	9,886	60.8	47,887	86.4
Alabama	3,324	82.7	1,989	95.7	151	59.7	299	59.0	68	43.9	817	79.6
Alaska	141	97.2	137	103.0	—	—	4	33.0	—	—	—	—
Arizona	1,414	87.8	501	98.2	96	75.6	219	88.3	29	65.9	569	83.6
Arkansas	1,060	74.0	227	64.1	—	—	138	80.2	94	55.0	601	81.8
California	14,464	81.7	6,290	87.5	1,586	77.1	1,837	76.1	1,150	77.5	3,601	79.0
Colorado	2,748	84.1	964	81.7	247	81.0	166	75.1	110	71.0	1,261	89.6
Connecticut	4,352	89.6	2,195	89.8	759	93.0	362	92.1	146	117.7	890	82.5
Delaware	691	89.5	611	90.8	44	88.0	10	66.7	3	75.0	23	76.7
Dist. of Col.	2,493	88.5	1,967	90.6	167	83.9	151	81.6	8	61.5	200	80.0
Florida	8,692	87.5	5,756	92.9	701	72.6	960	74.7	383	67.4	892	96.7
Georgia	6,196	78.7	4,301	86.9	551	85.0	372	62.3	340	52.9	632	61.0
Hawaii	274	71.4	151	75.9	—	—	32	52.5	48	64.9	43	86.0
Idaho	307	71.4	203	76.3	—	—	25	89.3	5	35.7	74	60.7
Illinois	9,364	89.3	4,121	85.7	521	83.1	1,936	102.1	491	76.4	2,295	91.4
Indiana	5,300	80.7	3,011	83.7	—	—	675	88.9	446	55.3	1,168	83.0
Iowa	2,582	79.1	1,142	79.7	—	—	554	79.3	103	45.6	783	86.3
Kansas	2,627	81.9	1,101	82.0	247	90.5	335	67.7	242	79.6	702	88.5
Kentucky	2,032	76.2	811	84.7	277	58.8	285	75.8	126	42.6	533	94.0
Louisiana	3,147	87.9	2,332	92.8	395	81.3	260	75.1	42	58.3	118	72.0
Maine	1,450	90.4	600	87.0	—	—	17	77.3	50	75.8	783	94.8
Maryland	5,389	83.5	3,751	83.6	652	94.4	99	37.4	124	77.5	763	89.6
Massachusetts	8,543	85.9	2,879	82.5	773	90.0	615	89.4	734	73.3	3,542	90.6

State												
Michigan	8,007	86.3	4,521	88.4	679	87.6	856	83.8	138	64.5	1,813	84.2
Minnesota	4,748	82.4	2,381	81.5	–	–	1,027	82.5	42	63.6	1,298	85.0
Mississippi	2,605	81.8	1,918	85.9	58	103.6	90	81.1	61	28.4	478	83.9
Missouri	4,893	81.1	3,060	86.8	93	93.0	726	84.8	334	48.0	680	79.6
Montana	479	68.2	373	79.5	–	–	11	19.6	15	18.5	80	83.3
Nebraska	1,009	77.7	671	81.1	–	–	171	72.8	52	47.7	115	89.8
Nevada	282	82.2	132	89.8	–	–	48	66.7	33	64.7	69	94.5
New Hampshire	764	97.0	517	104.7	55	98.2	23	74.2	38	53.5	131	96.3
New Jersey	8,274	83.7	6,208	90.0	438	95.2	340	41.1	301	77.4	987	75.6
New Mexico	535	88.0	323	100.9	55	59.8	21	75.0	56	68.3	80	93.0
New York	37,253	94.8	26,858	97.1	690	79.3	2,916	89.9	742	86.9	6,047	90.6
North Carolina	6,339	76.7	3,504	84.5	290	67.3	498	81.4	645	34.6	1,402	116.4
North Dakota	715	78.7	608	77.2	–	–	84	82.4	23	121.1	–	–
Ohio	10,634	80.1	5,855	83.4	460	81.9	1,775	87.3	427	63.0	2,117	70.9
Oklahoma	2,492	77.3	1,921	77.8	49	52.7	308	81.5	61	65.6	153	80.5
Oregon	1,639	81.8	992	83.5	41	64.1	183	73.5	5	62.5	418	84.4
Pennsylvania	17,025	84.5	10,203	82.3	1,129	86.9	927	72.1	747	82.5	4,019	94.3
Rhode Island	1,299	113.9	939	127.5	145	86.3	48	100.0	24	68.6	143	93.5
South Carolina	3,809	89.2	3,334	92.3	–	–	172	65.6	177	72.2	126	85.1
South Dakota	849	77.4	488	89.1	–	–	33	61.1	39	22.2	289	90.6
Tennessee	4,756	87.2	2,970	93.8	192	69.8	374	73.8	162	49.2	1,058	89.9
Texas	10,627	80.4	5,625	81.4	1,063	82.3	1,444	68.2	168	59.4	2,327	89.0
Utah	612	68.6	323	88.0	–	–	72	42.4	53	62.4	164	60.7
Vermont	610	93.3	362	96.0	123	104.2	26	81.3	29	60.4	70	88.6
Virginia	7,208	85.0	5,189	92.2	775	68.9	416	68.3	136	70.1	692	74.9
Washington	2,379	88.9	1,238	91.9	90	68.7	244	68.9	63	55.8	744	101.6
West Virginia	2,417	84.5	1,962	91.1	49	90.7	201	88.5	116	38.2	89	72.4
Wisconsin	3,954	77.4	844	84.0	260	84.1	725	77.6	449	46.1	1,676	88.7
Wyoming	581	68.8	241	66.0	–	–	–	–	8	13.6	332	79.0

Source: *National Institute of Mental Health.* Unpublished provisional estimates from the Survey and Reports Branch, Division of Biometry and Epidemiology.

Note: Information on facilities in Puerto Rico, Virgin Islands, and other U.S. territories are excluded.

*Since data for 1979 are *not* available for nonfederal general hospital psychiatric inpatient services, data are shown for 1977.

†Since data for 1979 are *not* available for federally funded community mental health centers, data are shown for 1980.

‡This category includes V.A. psychiatric services, residential treatment centers for emotionally disturbed children, and other multiservice mental health facilities with an inpatient setting which are *not* elsewhere classified.

**Since data for 1979 are *not* available for V.A. psychiatric services, data are shown for 1977.

TABLE 1–15. Average Daily Inpatient Census and Percentage Occupancy, by Type of Mental Health Facility: United States, selected years 1969–79

TYPE OF FACILITY	1969	1971	1973	1975	1977	1979
	Average daily inpatient census					
All facilities	468,831	420,930	346,233	287,588	252,304	233,384
State and county mental hospitals	367,629	326,575	252,630	193,380	156,729	138,600
Private psychiatric hospitals	11,608	11,562	11,255	12,058	13,129	13,901
Nonfederal general hospital psychiatric services	17,808	18,701	19,151	22,874	23,110	23,110*
V.A. psychiatric services†	47,140	39,115	35,575	32,123	28,693	28,693*
Federally funded community mental health centers	5,270	6,096	8,975	10,186	10,460	9,886*
Residential treatment centers for emotionally disturbed children	12,406	17,414	17,364	16,164	17,934	18,054
All other facilities‡	970	1,467	1,283	803	1,805	1,140
	Occupancy (%)					
All facilities	88.2	89.2	88.3	84.4	83.8	85.0
State and county mental hospitals	89.4	90.7	90.5	87.0	85.1	88.6
Private psychiatric hospitals	81.2	80.2	73.2	74.9	78.9	81.0
Nonfederal general hospital psychiatric services	79.5	80.3	78.2	79.7	78.6	78.6*
V.A. psychiatric services†	93.0	92.5	88.9	89.4	86.2	84.9*
Federally funded community mental health centers	65.0	57.8	72.4	59.8	70.6	60.8*
Residential treatment centers for emotionally disturbed children	82.0	90.0	91.3	89.7	89.4	89.4
All other facilities‡	81.0	82.1	81.2	80.9	81.0	79.6

Source: *National Institute of Mental Health.* Unpublished data from the Survey and Reports Branch, Division of Biometry and Epidemiology.

Note: See Table 1–2.

*Since data for 1979 are *not* available for V.A. psychiatric services, separate psychiatric services of nonfederal general hospitals, and federally funded community mental health centers (CMHCs), data are shown for 1980 for CMHCs and for 1977 for V.A. psychiatric services and separate psychiatric services of nonfederal general hospitals.

†Includes V.A. neuropsychiatric hospitals, V.A. general hospitals with separate psychiatric settings, and V.A. freestanding psychiatric outpatient clinics.

‡Includes other multiservice mental health facilities with an inpatient setting which are *not* elsewhere classified.

Primary-care physicians saw patients with neuroses other than depression more than any other type of mentally disturbed patient (Table 1—17).

The number of visits in which patients were treated with a psychotherapeutic listening treatment and the average duration of the visit in minutes are shown in Table 1–18. The longest sessions were those conducted by a psychiatrist, the shortest by a family physician and obstetrician/gynecologist.

When surveyed, Ph.D. psychologists reported that the problem they treated most was a marital or family problem. The least common patient problem in their practice was mental retardation, followed closely by sexual assault. Therapists with master's de-

TABLE 1–17. Percentage Distribution of Office Visits with a Principal Diagnosis of Mental Disorder by Diagnostic Category, in Psychiatry and Primary Care: United States, 1980

PRINCIPAL DIAGNOSES OF MENTAL DISORDER	PHYSICIAN SPECIALTY		
	All specialties	Psychiatry	Primary care
Number of visits (in 000s)	24,343	14,735	8,125
Percent	100.0	100.0	100.0
Alcohol and drug-related disorders	3.1	–	5.9
Affective disorders	23.8	27.6	19.0
Schizophrenia and related disorders	7.2	10.8	–
Neuroses other than depressive	28.3	18.5	42.2
Personality disorders	9.4	15.3	–
Other mental disorders	28.4	26.4	31.0

Source: *National Institute of Mental Health.* Compiled from unpublished data from the National Ambulatory Medical Care Survey.

TABLE 1–18. Percentage Distribution of Office Visits with a Psychotherapy/Psychotherapeutic Listening Treatment, Percent of All Office Visits, and Mean Duration of Office Visits with Such Treatments, According to Physician Specialty: United States, 1980

PHYSICIAN SPECIALTY	VISITS WITH A PSYCHOTHERAPY/ PSYCHOTHERAPEUTIC LISTENING TREATMENT		
	Percentage distribution (N=29,024,000)	As percentage of all visits to physician specialty	Mean duration of visit (minutes)
All specialties	100.0	5.0	33
Psychiatry	50.7	92.8	45
Family/general practice	15.8 ⎫	2.4 ⎫	17 ⎫
Internal medicine	12.7 ⎬ 49.4	5.3 ⎬ 2.6	24 ⎬ 21
Pediatrics	3.9 ⎪	1.8 ⎪	19 ⎪
Obstetrics/gynecology	6.8 ⎪	3.6 ⎪	16 ⎪
Other specialties	10.2 ⎭	1.6 ⎭	25 ⎭

Source: *National Institute of Mental Health.* Compiled from unpublished data from the National Ambulatory Medical Care Survey.

grees most often treated patients with school problems. Those least commonly treated were sexual-assault victims.

The employment settings in which mental health service providers trained in psychology typically work were reported. According to surveys conducted by the American Psychological Association, 20% of doctoral-level professionals work in their own private practice; those with a master's degree worked in a community mental health center setting.

The number of full-time equivalent positions in various kinds of facilities in 1978 are presented in Table 1–19. Positions classified as "other patient care staff," mental health care workers with less than a B.A. degree, and clerical workers comprise the largest components of the full-time positions in mental health.

The supply of professionals with Ph.D. degrees in psychology since 1958 has increased yearly at a steady rate (Table 1–20).

Similarly, the psychiatry residencies filled yearly in the United States between 1961 and 1981 have increased greatly, from 29,494

TABLE 1–19. Full-time Equivalent Positions in Mental Health Facilities, by Facility and Staff Discipline: United States, 1978

| | | PSYCHIATRIC HOSPITAL | | |
STAFF DISCIPLINE	All facilities	Total	State and county mental hospitals	Private psychiatric hospitals
All staff	430,051	235,261	205,289	29,972
Professional patient care staff	153,598	56,550	45,131	11,419
Psychiatrists	14,492	4,997	3,712	1,285
Other physicians	3,034	1,994	1,809	185
Psychologists	16,501	3,739	3,149	590
Masters and above	14,814	3,244	2,690	554
Doctorate	7,986	1,612	1,197	415
Masters	6,828	1,632	1,493	139
Other psychologists	1,687	495	459	36
Social workers	28,125	6,844	5,924	920
MSW (or MA) and above	21,238	4,141	3,373	768
Other social workers	6,887	2,703	2,551	152
Registered nurses	42,399	18,826	14,859	3,967
Other mental health professionals – BA and above (e.g., vocational rehabilitation counselors, occupational therapists, and teachers)	39,363	14,136	10,492	3,644
Physical health professionals and assistants (e.g., dentists, dental technicians, pharmacists, and dieticians)	9,684	6,014	5,186	828
Other patient care staff	139,101	93,365	86,056	7,309
Licensed practical or vocational nurses	16,587	9,521	8,323	1,198
Mental health workers (less than BA)	122,514	83,844	77,733	6,111
All other staff	137,352	85,346	74,102	11,244
Administrative and other professional (nonhealth) staff (e.g., accountants and business administrators)	12,962	4,828	3,489	1,339
Other staff (clerical and maintenance)	124,390	80,518	70,613	9,905

continued

TABLE 1–19. Continued

STAFF DISCIPLINE	NON-FEDERAL GENERAL HOSPITAL PSYCHIATRIC SERVICES Total	Inpatient units	Outpatient units	VETERANS ADMINISTRATION PSYCHIATRIC SERVICES Total	Neuropsychiatric hospitals	General hospital inpatient	General hospital outpatient
All staff	40,908	33,842	7,066	41,449	24,761	14,613	2,075
Professional patient care staff	22,401	17,254	5,147	15,238	7,266	6,447	1,525
Psychiatrists	3,583	1,779	1,804	1,745	335	1,040	370
Other physicians	237	167	70	509	342	144	23
Psychologists	1,512	565	947	1,392	367	664	361
Masters and above	1,392	520	872	1,259	317	600	342
Doctorate	946	381	565	1,073	290	487	296
Masters	446	139	307	186	27	113	46
Other psychologists	120	45	75	133	50	64	19
Social workers	2,552	1,149	1,403	1,611	652	564	395
MSW (or MA) and above	2,114	895	1,219	1,404	551	499	354
Other social workers	438	254	184	207	101	65	41
Registered nurses	10,611	10,250	361	5,814	2,983	2,673	158
Other mental health professionals – BA and above (e.g., vocational rehabilitation counselors, occupational therapists, and teachers)	3,583	3,071	512	1,868	1,026	725	101
Physical health professionals and assistants (e.g., dentists, dental technicians, pharmacists, and dieticians)	323	273	50	2,299	1,561	637	117
Other patient care staff	12,565	12,289	276	12,197	7,847	4,239	111
Licensed practical or vocational nurses	3,395	3,354	41	1,751	1,032	703	95
Mental health workers (less than BA)	9,170	8,935	235	10,446	6,815	3,536	16
All other staff	5,942	4,299	1,643	14,014	9,648	3,927	439
Administrative and other professional (nonhealth) staff (e.g., accountants and business administrators)	452	274	178	1,366	872	435	59
Other staff (clerical and maintenance)	5,490	4,025	1,465	12,648	8,776	3,492	380

Source: *Mental Health, United States 1983*

in 1961 to 67,868 in 1981 (Table 1–21).

The cost of mental health care in 1980 was greatest for general hospital psychiatric services (Figure 1–4).

The total expenditures and per capita expenditures in current dollars by type of mental health facility are shown in Table 1–22. The per capita cost in state and county mental hospitals was $16.86 as of 1979. The same cost in community mental health centers was $6.65.

TABLE 1–20. Trends in the Psychology Doctoral Degrees Awarded and Percent in Selected Subfields: United States, 1958–81

ACADEMIC YEAR	PSYCHOLOGY DOCTORATES	CLINICAL		COUNSELING	
		Number	Percent	Number	Percent
1957–1958	745	246	33.0	45	6.0
1958–1959	787	283	36.0	46	5.8
1959–1960	773	241	31.2	67	8.7
1960–1961	820	299	36.5	67	8.2
1961–1962	857	293	34.2	60	7.0
1962–1963	892	303	34.0	48	5.4
1963–1964	1,013	398	39.3	47	4.6
1964–1965	955	335	35.1	47	4.9
1965–1966	1,133	368	32.5	57	5.0
1966–1967	1,293	417	32.3	79	6.1
1967–1968	1,452	483	33.3	103	7.1
1968–1969	1,728	525	30.4	108	6.2
1969–1970	1,883	549	29.2	113	6.0
1970–1971	2,116	616	29.1	144	6.8
1971–1972	2,262	671	29.7	151	6.7
1972–1973	2,444	737	30.2	199	8.1
1973–1974	2,587	751	29.0	208	8.0
1974–1975	2,749	811	29.5	231	8.4
1975–1976	2,878	881	30.6	266	9.2
1976–1977	2,960	914	30.9	263	8.9
1977–1978	3,049	1,066	35.0	272	8.9
1978–1979	3,081	1,056	34.3	315	10.2
1979–1980	3,098	1,106	35.7	298	9.6
1980–1981	3,357	1,256	37.4	351	10.5

Source: *National Research Council. Summary Report: Doctorate Recipients from United States Universities.* Washington, D.C.: National Academy Press, 1981 and previous years.

TABLE 1–21. Filled Psychiatry Residencies as a Percentage of Total Filled Residencies and Percent Filled by Foreign Medical Graduates: United States, 1961–81

YEAR*	TOTAL RESIDENCIES FILLED	PSYCHIATRY AND CHILD PSYCHIATRY RESIDENCIES FILLED		PERCENTAGE OF RESIDENCIES FILLED BY FOREIGN MEDICAL GRADUATES	
		Number	As a percentage of total	Total residencies	Psychiatry and child psychiatry residencies
1961	29,494	3,428	11.6	–	–
1962	29,053	3,488	12.0	–	–
1963	29,295	3,617	12.3	24.1	23.2
1964	30,797	3,804	12.4	26.4	24.3
1965	31,687	3,899	12.3	28.8	26.2
1966	31,792	3,922	12.3	29.8	26.4
1967	33,509	4,061	12.1	31.6	27.8
1968	34,794	4,093	11.8	32.2	28.3
1969	36,492	4,003	11.0	33.0	30.1
1970	39,220	4,295	11.0	33.0	27.2
1971	42,293	4,613	10.9	32.0	26.7
1972	44,858	4,641	10.3	32.2	27.2
1973	48,869	4,903	10.0	30.5	29.9
1974	52,499	4,940	9.4	29.3	35.2
1975	NA	NA	–	–	–
1976	60,318	4,938	8.2	25.6	34.5
1977†	56,019	4,485	8.0	24.5	33.6
1978	63,163	4,608	7.3	20.3	30.0
1979	64,615	4,422	6.8	18.7	27.0
1980	61,819	4,337	7.0	19.5	28.6
1981	67,868	4,823	7.1	19.4	29.2

Source: *American Medical Association. Directory of Residency Training Programs.* Chicago, Ill.: the Association, 1982 and previous years.
*As of September 1
†86% response rate

FIG. 1–4. Estimates of direct costs of mental health care: health and specialty mental health sectors United States–1980

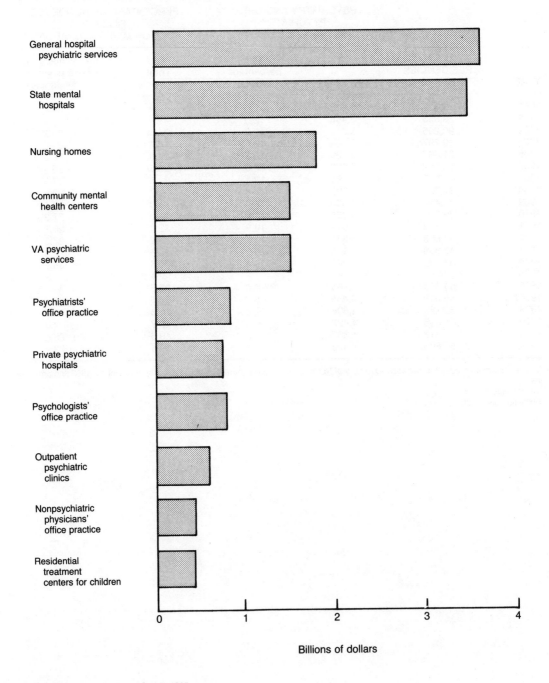

Billions of dollars

Source: *MentalHealth*, United States 1985

TABLE 1–22. Total Expenditures in Current Dollars, Percentage Distribution, and Per Capita Expenditures, by Type of Mental Health Facility: United States, selected years 1969–79

TYPE OF FACILITY	1969	1971	1973	1975	1977	1979
	Total expenditures in thousands of dollars					
All facilities	3,292,563	4,284,700	5,085,528	6,564,312	7,463,000	8,763,795
State and county mental hospitals	1,814,101	2,359,000	2,574,803	3,185,049	3,330,249	3,756,754
Private psychiatric hospitals	220,026	276,000	328,463	466,720	563,294	743,037
Nonfederal general hospital psychiatric services	298,000	373,000	450,715	621,284	722,868	722,868
V.A. psychiatric services†	450,000	500,000	624,257	699,027	848,469	848,469
Federally funded community mental health centers	143,491	294,000	468,658	775,580	990,199	1,480,890
Residential treatment centers for emotionally disturbed children	122,711	197,000	245,995	278,950	359,060	436,246
Freestanding psychiatric outpatient clinics	185,517	209,000	301,758	421,557	493,314	588,690
All other facilities‡	58,717	76,700	90,879	116,145	155,547	186,841
	Percentage distribution of total expenditures					
All facilities	100.0	100.0	100.0	100.0	100.0	100.0
State and county mental hospitals	55.1	55.0	50.6	48.5	44.6	42.9
Private psychiatric hospitals	6.7	6.4	6.5	7.1	7.5	8.5
Nonfederal general hospital psychiatric services	9.0	8.7	8.9	9.5	9.7	8.2*
V.A. psychiatric services†	13.7	11.7	12.3	10.6	11.4	9.7*
Federally funded community mental health centers	4.4	6.9	9.2	11.8	13.3	6.9*
Residential treatment centers for emotionally disturbed children	3.7	4.6	4.8	4.3	4.8	5.0
Freestanding psychiatric outpatient clinics	5.6	4.9	5.9	6.4	6.6	6.7
All other facilities‡	1.8	1.8	1.8	1.8	2.1	2.1
	Per capita expenditures**					
All facilities	$16.53	$20.97	$24.44	$31.05	$34.76	$39.61
State and county mental hospitals	9.11	11.55	12.37	15.06	15.51	16.86
Private psychiatric hospitals	1.10	1.35	1.58	2.21	2.62	3.34
Nonfederal general hospital psychiatric services	1.50	1.83	2.17	2.94	3.37	3.37*
V.A. psychiatric services†	2.26	2.45	3.00	3.31	3.95	3.95*
Federally funded community mental health centers	.72	1.44	2.25	3.67	4.61	6.65*
Residential treatment centers for emotionally disturbed children	.62	.96	1.18	1.32	1.67	1.96
Freestanding psychiatric outpatient clinics	.93	1.02	1.45	1.99	2.30	2.64
All other facilities‡	.29	.37	.44	.55	.73	.84

Source: *National Institute of Mental Health.* Unpublished data from the Survey and Reports Branch, Division of Biometry and Epidemiology.

Notes: See Table 1–2.

*Based on the medical care component of the consumer price index (1969 = 100.0). Indices for other years are 1971 (113.2); 1973 (121.4); 1975 (148.7); 1977 (178.5); and 1979 (211.4).

†Since 1979 data are *not* available for V.A. psychiatric services, separate psychiatric services of nonfederal general hospitals, and federally funded community mental health centers (CMHCs), data are shown for 1980 for CMHCs and for 1977 for V.A. psychiatric services and separate psychiatric services of nonfederal general hospitals.

‡Includes V.A. neuropsychiatric hospitals, V.A. general hospitals with separate psychiatric settings, and V.A. freestanding psychiatric outpatient clinics.

**Includes freestanding psychiatric day/night facilities and other multiservice mental health facilities with an inpatient setting which are *not* elsewhere classified.

¶The population used in the calculation of these rates is the civilian population of the United States for each year as provided by the Bureau of the Census and published in Series P-25 publications.

2 Forms of Mental Disease

Much information has been collected on the utilization of mental health resources defined in terms of admission rates, treatment episodes, psychiatric beds, and patient: staff ratios. But epidemiologic studies on the incidence and prevalence of mental disorders in the U.S. population overall are scanty. Where studies exist, results of diagnostic counts are difficult to compare because studies often use different diagnostic criteria. But in late 1984, data from a major national effort sponsored by the National Institutes of Mental Health (NIMH) using the Diagnostic and Statistical Manual of Mental Disorders (DSM III) were gathered and analyzed. The study was the largest of any undertaken in North America. It surveyed 17,000 community residents in five epidemiologic catchment areas (EPAs) including Baltimore, New Haven, North Carolina, St. Louis, and Los Angeles. Subjects were interviewed through use of a Diagnostic Interview Schedule (DIS), a structured interview instrument that lay personnel were able to administer.

PREVALENCE

This research is regarded as a hallmark in the study of mental disease. Unlike previous U.S. studies, it assesses untreated illness and the number of past episodes of mental illness as well as current

36

ones among persons surveyed. The large sample size has enabled researchers to study all the diagnoses of the DSM III classification including low-frequency disorders. In addition, the DIS has been translated and is therefore a field instrument that can be used for cross-cultural comparison studies.

The preliminary results of this study confirmed estimates from smaller studies. The latter indicated that 17% to 23% of adults have had at least one mental disorder. The rates of the often-neglected disorders triggered by substance abuse were estimated at between 6% and 7%. The rate of affective (depressive) disorders was 5% to 6%; anxiety diagnoses were as high as 7% to 15%. Only 23% of anxiety disorders were treated and only one-half of schizophren-ics had ever been treated.

The lifetime prevalence of the 15 major mental disorders studied was determined by asking respondents whether they had ever had each symptom that serves as a criterion for the disease. The respondent was also probed for the severity of the symptom and its nonphysical cause. A maximum age of onset was additionally required for some disorders, such as schizophrenia, as was a minimum frequency of episodes for other syndromes, such as panic disorder.

Investigators also studied the rate of recall among those known to have been treated years earlier for hallucinations or delusions. The rate of recall prompted by a DIS session was 85% for delusional subjects and 64% for those who had hallucinated. These high rates were found even though not all of the subjects were in remission. The problem of recall bias was thus addressed; however, it contin-ued to elicit cautious analysis of the data by researchers even though the tested recall among formerly treated patients was sufficient to differentiate them from those in the general popula-tion reporting these symptoms at a rate of only 4% to 5%.

Those who had experienced at least one mental disorder during their lifetime varied from 28.8% in New Haven to 38.0% in Baltimore (Table 2–1). The rate between Baltimore, New Haven, and St. Louis was significantly different; it derived mainly from a higher rate of phobias reported in Baltimore. The most common disorders were alcohol abuse (11% and 16%) followed by drug abuse (5% and 6%). The data across the various sites indicate that one in 20 persons suffers at least one major depressive disorder at some time in his or her life; one in 30 suffers dysthymia, and one in 40 has had an antisocial personality or an obsessive compulsive disorder. Less than one in 50 persons developed a panic disorder, cognitive impairment, or schizophrenia. Anorexia nervosa, somatization disorder, and schizophreniform disorder all occurred in one in 500 persons in each EPA.

TABLE 2–1. Sex Predominance of Disorders Across Sites*

PROBLEM	NEW HAVEN, CONN. (%)		BALTIMORE (%)		ST. LOUIS (%)	
	M N=1,292	F N=1,766	M N=1,322	F N=2,159	M N=1,202	F N=1,802
Male predominant						
Definite:						
Antisocial personality	3.8 (0.6)	0.5 (0.2)†	4.9 (0.7)	0.7 (0.2)†	4.9 (0.7)	1.2 (0.3)†
Alcohol abuse/dependence	19.1 (1.1)	4.8 (0.5)†	24.9 (1.4)	4.2 (0.4)†	28.9 (1.8)	4.3 (0.6)†
Probable:						
Drug abuse/dependence	6.5 (0.7)	5.1 (0.6)	7.1 (0.8)	4.4 (0.6)‡	7.4 (0.9)	3.8 (0.6)†
Female predominant						
Definite:						
Major depressive episode	4.4 (0.6)	8.7 (0.8)†	2.3 (0.4)	4.9 (0.5)†	2.5 (0.5)	8.1 (0.9)†
Agoraphobia	1.5 (0.4)	5.3 (0.5)†	5.2 (0.6)	12.5 (1.0)†	1.5 (0.3)	6.4 (0.8)†
Simple phobia	3.8 (0.5)	8.5 (0.7)†	14.5 (1.1)	25.9 (1.2)†	4.0 (0.7)	9.4 (0.9)†
Probable						
Dysthymia	2.6 (0.5)	3.7 (0.4)	1.2 (0.3)	2.9 (0.4)†	2.1 (0.6)	5.4 (0.7)†
Somatization disorder	0.0 (0.0)	0.3 (0.1)‡	0.0 (0.0)	0.2 (0.1)**	0.0 (0.0)	0.3 (0.1)‡
Panic disorder	0.6 (0.2)	2.1 (0.4)†	1.2 (0.3)	1.6 (0.3)	0.9 (0.3)	2.0 (0.5)
Obsessive-compulsive	2.0 (0.4)	3.1 (0.4)	2.6 (0.6)	3.3 (0.5)	1.1 (0.3)	2.6 (0.5)‡
Schizophrenia	1.2 (0.3)	2.6 (0.4)‡	1.2 (0.3)	1.9 (0.3)	1.0 (0.4)	1.1 (0.3)
No predominance						
Manic episode	0.9 (0.3)	1.3 (0.3)	0.8 (0.3)	0.5 (0.2)	1.1 (0.4)	1.1 (0.3)
Cognitive impairment	1.4 (0.3)	1.2 (0.3)	1.1 (0.2)	1.4 (0.2)	1.0 (0.2)	1.1 (0.2)
Any of the covered diagnoses	30.6 (1.3)	27.3 (1.3)	39.6 (1.3)	36.7 (1.4)	37.0 (1.9)	25.7 (1.4)†

*Numbers in parentheses are SEs.
†P<.001
‡P<.01
**P<.05
Source: Robins JS, Helzer JE et al: Lifetime prevalence of specific psychiatric disorders in three sites. *Arch Gen Psychiat* 41 (10): 1984.

Six-month prevalence rates of the DSM III disorders (whether the disorder was present in a subject during a six-month period just prior to the survey) at the same three ECAs in 1980 were as would be expected, i.e., lower than the lifetime prevalence rates (Table 2–2).

Differences among the sites might be explained by age differences in the site populations, since mental disorders seem to occur in highest proportion among those age 25 to 44 years. But the sites reflected comparable age distributions.

Table 2–3 presents the lifetime prevalence rate for major DSM III disorders by age. At each of the three sites, persons age 25 to 44 years showed the highest prevalence rates for any covered diagnosis. The reason why younger people have a higher lifetime prevalence of mental disorders than older ones is puzzling. The reason may be a genuine change in the risk for more recent generations, or

TABLE 2-2. Six-Month Prevalence Rates of DIS/DSM III Disorders, Three ECA Sites*

DISORDERS	NEW HAVEN, CONN. % 1980–1981 (N=3,058)	BALTIMORE % 1981–1982 (N=3,481)	ST. LOUIS % 1981–1982 (N=3,004)
Any DIS disorder covered	18.4 (0.8)	23.4 (1.0)	16.8 (1.0)
Any DIS disorder except phobia	15.2 (0.8)	14.0 (0.7)	13.8 (0.9)
Any DIS disorder except substance use disorders	13.6 (0.7)	19.0 (0.9)	12.6 (0.9)
Substance use disorders:	6.1 (0.4)	7.2 (0.6)	5.8 (0.5)
Alcohol abuse/dependence	4.8 (0.4)	5.7 (0.6)	4.5 (0.5)
Drug abuse/dependence	1.8 (0.3)	2.2 (0.3)	2.0 (0.3)
Schizophrenic/schizophreniform disorders	1.1 (0.2)	1.2 (0.2)	0.6 (0.2)
Schizophrenia	1.1 (0.2)	1.0 (0.2)	0.6 (0.2)
Schizophreniform disorder	0.1 (0.1)	0.2 (0.1)	0.1 (0.0)
Affective disorders	6.5 (0.6)	4.6 (0.4)	6.2 (0.6)
Manic episode	0.8 (0.2)	0.4 (0.1)	0.7 (0.2)
Major depression	3.5 (0.4)	2.2 (0.3)	3.2 (0.5)
Dysthymia	3.2 (0.4)	2.1 (0.2)	3.8 (0.4)
Anxiety/somatoform disorders	7.2 (0.4)	14.9 (0.8)	6.6 (0.6)
Phobia	5.9 (0.4)	13.4 (0.8)	5.4 (0.5)
Panic	0.5 (0.1)	1.0 (0.2)	0.9 (0.2)
Obsessive-compulsive	1.4 (0.2)	2.0 (0.3)	1.3 (0.3)
Somatization	0.1 (0.1)	0.1 (0.1)	0.1 (0.1)
Personality disorder			
Antisocial personality	0.6 (0.1)	0.7 (0.2)	1.3 (0.3)
Cognitive impairment (severe)	1.3 (0.2)	1.3 (0.2)	1.0 (0.2)

*DIS indicates Diagnostic Interview Schedule; ECA, Epidemiologic Catchment Area; numbers in parentheses indicate SEs.
Source: Myers JK, Weissman MM, Tischler GL et al: Six-month prevalence of psychiatric disorders in three communities. *Arch Gen Psychiat* 41 (10): 1984.

TABLE 2–3. Lifetime Prevalence of *DSM III* Disorders by Age Group*

PROBLEM	NEW HAVEN, CONN. (%)				BALTIMORE (%)				ST. LOUIS (%)			
	1 N=422	2 N=1,277	3 N=785	4 N=607	1 N=504	2 N=1,212	3 N=842	4 N=923	1 N=471	2 N=1,233	3 N=724	4 N=576
Sites consistent: age group with highest rate												
25–44 yr:												
Schizophrenia	2.7	2.7	1.1	0.7	0.6	2.1	0.0	0.0	0.2	1.2	0.6	0.0
Panic	0.7	2.4	1.2	0.2	1.2	2.1	1.5	0.1	0.9	2.2	1.8	0.1
Obsessive-compulsive	2.8	3.8	1.5	1.3	3.5	3.9	2.5	1.2	2.2	2.4	1.4	1.1
Major depressive episode	7.5	10.4	4.2	1.8	4.1	7.5	4.2	1.4	4.5	8.0	5.2	0.8
Antisocial personality	2.7	3.1	1.1	0.8	2.1	4.5	1.9	0.4	4.3	5.2	1.4	0.2
18–24 yr:												
Drug abuse/dependence	17.5	7.2	0.6	0.1	12.0	9.0	0.6	0.0	11.0	8.3	0.6	0.1
Schizophreniform disorder	0.3	0.0	0.0	0.0	0.6	0.3	0.2	0.1	0.4	0.1	0.0	0.0
65+ yr:												
Cognitive impairment	0.5	0.3	1.1	5.0	0.2	0.3	1.1	5.1	0.7	0.2	0.7	4.0
Not consistent in all sites												
Anorexia nervosa	0.0	0.1	0.0	0.0	0.2	0.1	0.0	0.0	0.0	0.2	0.0	0.0
Manic episode	2.1	1.7	0.5	0.0	0.1	1.5	0.4	0.0	1.7	1.6	0.4	0.1
Somatization	0.1	0.3	0.1	0.0	0.0	0.2	0.0	0.0	0.3	0.1	0.1	0.0
Alcohol abuse/dependence	15.7	14.8	8.8	4.1	8.1	17.4	15.8	8.3	17.0	21.0	11.7	7.2
Agoraphobia	3.5	4.5	3.4	1.6	7.9	9.8	10.3	7.5	4.3	4.5	5.0	1.2
Simple phobia	5.0	7.4	6.4	4.6	21.0	21.1	21.5	18.1	5.8	8.7	6.7	3.5
Dysthymia	2.6	4.1	2.5	2.6	0.7	2.9	2.8	1.1	2.9	4.4	5.1	1.2
Any covered diagnosis	34.7	35.8	22.2	18.7	39.0	43.8	36.4	28.5	32.1	39.7	25.2	16.6

*Age codes are as follows: 1=18–24 yr; 2=25–44 yr; 3=45–64 yr; and 4=65+ yr.
Source: See Table 2–1.

disorder-related mortality, which decreases the number of people still living at advanced age who have had the disorder. Again, it may simply be the result of less accurate recall among older respondents.

The disorders occurring most often in the younger age groups are shown in Table 2–4.

Certain disorders were also sex predominant. Alcohol abuse or dependence and antisocial personality were much more prevalent in men at all three sites; depression, agoraphobia, and simple phobia were much more common in women. Cognitive impairment showed no pattern by sex (Table 2–5).

The lifetime prevalence of DSM III diagnoses by race is presented in Table 2–6. The major difference between white and nonwhite respondents appears to be in the lifetime prevalence of phobia. The population of Baltimore had three times as many blacks as that of New Haven. This fact may in part explain why the report of phobia was more common in Baltimore. However, whites in Baltimore also reported a higher lifetime prevalence of phobia. Differences between the races for other diagnoses were not statistically significant.

New Haven had the greatest proportion of college graduates reporting a mental disorder in their lifetime; Baltimore had the lowest. However, more Baltimoreans reported phobia among both the educated and noneducated (Table 2–7).

TABLE 2–4. Disorders with Significantly High Prevalence in Younger Age Groups*

	SIGNIFICANT AGE COMPARISONS IN THREE SITES (in years)		
DISORDER	18–24 25–44	25–44 45–64	45–64 65+
Major depressive episode	0	3	3
Manic episode	0	3	3
Alcohol abuse or dependence	0	2	3
Drug abuse or dependence	1	3	1
Antisocial personality	0	3	2
Agoraphobia	0	1	2
Panic disorder	0	0	3
Schizophrenia	0	2	0
Dysthymia	0	0	2
Simple phobia	0	0	1
Total	1	17	20

*None significant: cognitive deficit, obsessive-compulsive disorder, somatization disorder, anorexia nervosa, and schizophreniform disorder.
Source: See Table 2–1.

Except for panic syndrome, most mental disorders were more prevalent among inner city respondents. This may not necessarily indicate the effects of inner city life on mental health; it may reflect in part the fact that those with untreated problems tend to gravitate to the inner city where community services, support groups, and anonymity are more readily available than in rural areas.

TABLE 2–5. Sex Predominance of Disorders Across Sites*

PROBLEM	NEW HAVEN, CONN. (%)		BALTIMORE (%)		ST. LOUIS (%)	
	M N=1,292	F N=1,766	M N=1,322	F N=2,159	M N=1,202	F N=1,802
Male predominant						
Definite:						
Antisocial personality	3.8 (0.6)	0.5 (0.2)†	4.9 (0.7)	0.7 (0.2)†	4.9 (0.7)	1.2 (0.3)†
Alcohol abuse/dependence	19.1 (1.1)	4.8 (0.5)†	24.9 (1.4)	4.2 (0.4)†	28.9 (1.8)	4.3 (0.6)†
Probable:						
Drug abuse/dependence	6.5 (0.7)	5.1 (0.6)	7.1 (0.8)	4.4 (0.6)‡	7.4 (0.9)	3.8 (0.6)†
Female predominant						
Definite:						
Major depressive episode	4.4 (0.6)	8.7 (0.8)†	2.3 (0.4)	4.9 (0.5)†	2.5 (0.5)	8.1 (0.9)†
Agoraphobia	1.5 (0.4)	5.3 (0.5)†	5.2 (0.6)	12.5 (1.0)†	1.5 (0.3)	6.4 (0.8)†
Simple phobia	3.8 (0.5)	8.5 (0.7)†	14.5 (1.1)	25.9 (1.2)†	4.0 (0.7)	9.4 (0.9)†
Probable						
Dysthymia	2.6 (0.5)	3.7 (0.4)	1.2 (0.3)	2.9 (0.4)†	2.1 (0.6)	5.4 (0.7)†
Somatization disorder	0.0 (0.0)	0.3 (0.1)‡	0.0 (0.0)	0.2 (0.1)**	0.0 (0.0)	0.3 (0.1)‡
Panic disorder	0.6 (0.2)	2.1 (0.4)†	1.2 (0.3)	1.6 (0.3)	0.9 (0.3)	2.0 (0.5)
Obsessive-compulsive	2.0 (0.4)	3.1 (0.4)	2.6 (0.6)	3.3 (0.5)	1.1 (0.3)	2.6 (0.5)‡
Schizophrenia	1.2 (0.3)	2.6 (0.4)‡	1.2 (0.3)	1.9 (0.3)	1.0 (0.4)	1.1 (0.3)
No predominance						
Manic episode	0.9 (0.3)	1.3 (0.3)	0.8 (0.3)	0.5 (0.2)	1.1 (0.4)	1.1 (0.3)
Cognitive impairment	1.4 (0.3)	1.2 (0.3)	1.1 (0.2)	1.4 (0.2)	1.0 (0.2)	1.1 (0.2)
Any of the covered diagnoses	30.6 (1.3)	27.3 (1.3)	39.6 (1.3)	36.7 (1.4)	37.0 (1.9)	25.7 (1.4)†

*Numbers in parentheses are SEs.
†P<.001
‡P<.01
**P<.05
Source: See Table 2–1.

TABLE 2–6. Lifetime Prevalence of *DSM-III* Diagnoses by Race*

	NEW HAVEN, CONN. (%)		BALTIMORE (%)		ST. LOUIS (%)	
	Black N=334	Nonblack N=2,708	Black N=1,182	Nonblack N=2,299	Black N=1,158	Nonblack N=1,846
Simple phobias	5.1 (1.6)	6.4 (0.5)	27.6 (1.4)	17.4 (1.1)†	11.1 (1.2)	5.9 (0.7)†
Agoraphobia	4.4 (1.0)	3.4 (0.3)	13.4 (1.2)	7.2 (0.7)†	4.4 (0.7)	4.1 (0.6)
Drug abuse/dependence	6.4 (1.3)	5.7 (0.5)	7.3 (0.9)	4.9 (0.5)‡	6.4 (1.0)	5.3 (0.7)
Cognitive impairment	1.9 (0.6)	1.3 (0.2)	1.8 (0.3)	1.1 (0.2)	2.2 (0.3)	0.7 (0.2)†
Schizophrenia	2.1 (0.7)	1.9 (0.3)	2.4 (0.5)	1.2 (0.2)‡	1.0 (0.3)	1.0 (0.3)
Manic episode	1.0 (0.5)	1.2 (0.2)	0.5 (0.2)	0.7 (0.2)	2.5 (0.8)	0.7 (0.2)‡
Somatization	0.7 (0.4)	0.1 (0.0)	0.1 (0.1)	0.1 (0.1)	0.4 (0.2)	0.1 (0.1)
Major depressive episode	5.7 (1.5)	6.8 (0.5)	3.7 (0.7)	3.8 (0.4)	4.9 (0.8)	5.7 (0.7)
Anorexia nervosa	0.0 (0.0)	0.1 (0.0)	0.0 (0.0)	0.1 (0.1)	0.0 (0.0)	0.1 (0.1)
Schizophreniform disorder	0.0 (0.0)	0.1 (0.1)	0.4 (0.2)	0.3 (0.1)	0.0 (0.0)	0.1 (0.1)
Dysthymia	3.3 (1.1)	3.2 (0.4)	1.8 (0.5)	2.3 (0.3)	3.6 (0.7)	3.9 (0.5)
Panic	1.3 (0.6)	1.5 (0.2)	1.6 (0.4)	1.3 (0.2)	1.1 (0.3)	1.6 (0.4)
Obsessive-compulsive	2.7 (0.8)	2.6 (0.3)	2.7 (0.5)	3.1 (0.4)	1.5 (0.4)	2.0 (0.4)
Alcohol abuse/dependence	14.3 (2.4)	11.1 (0.6)	14.6 (1.1)	13.2 (0.8)	14.7 (1.6)	16.0 (1.1)
Antisocial personality	1.7 (0.6)	2.1 (0.3)	2.3 (0.5)	2.7 (0.4)	3.9 (0.9)	3.1 (0.5)
Any of the covered diagnoses	30.5 (3.1)	28.6 (1.0)	45.1 (1.8)	34.7 (1.1)†	34.9 (1.9)	30.1 (1.4)‡

*Numbers in parentheses are SEs
†P<.001
‡P<.05
Source: See Table 2–1.

TABLE 2–7. Lifetime Prevalence of *DSM-III* Diagnoses by Education*

	NEW HAVEN, CONN. (%)		BALTIMORE (%)		ST. LOUIS (%)	
PROBLEM	College Graduate N=839	Other N=2,218	College Graduate N=303	Other N=3,174	College Graduate N=416	Other N=2,496
Cognitive impairment	0.3 (0.2)	1.7 (0.3)†	0.2 (0.2)	1.4 (0.2)†	0.0 (0.0)	0.8 (0.1)†
Simple phobia	3.8 (0.8)	7.2 (0.5)†	12.8 (2.3)	21.4 (0.9)‡	5.1 (1.5)	7.2 (0.7)
Agoraphobia	2.2 (0.5)	4.1 (0.4)**	4.4 (1.1)	9.6 (0.6)†	2.1 (0.8)	4.5 (0.5)**
Schizophrenia	0.5 (0.3)	2.5 (0.3)†	0.6 (0.4)	1.7 (0.3)	0.6 (0.3)	1.1 (0.3)
Schizophreniform disorder	0.0 (0.0)	0.1 (0.1)	0.0 (0.0)	0.3 (0.1)†	0.0 (0.0)	0.1 (0.1)
Alcohol abuse/dependence	5.5 (1.0)	12.2 (0.8)**	12.1 (2.4)	13.8 (0.7)	15.3 (2.3)	15.9 (1.0)
Somatization	0.0 (0.0)	0.2 (0.1)**	0.0 (0.0)	0.1 (0.1)	0.1 (0.1)	0.2 (0.1)
Panic	1.6 (0.4)	1.4 (0.3)	1.1 (0.6)	1.5 (0.2)	0.5 (0.3)	1.7 (0.4)**
Manic episode	0.7 (0.3)	1.3 (0.3)	0.3 (0.3)	0.7 (0.2)	0.6 (0.4)	1.1 (0.3)
Antisocial personality	0.9 (0.4)	2.5 (0.4)	1.5 (0.8)	2.7 (0.3)	2.3 (1.0)	3.4 (0.5)
Major depressive episode	7.1 (1.1)	6.6 (0.5)	5.5 (1.2)	3.6 (0.3)	4.6 (0.9)	5.7 (0.6)
Dysthymia	2.2 (0.6)	3.5 (0.4)	2.5 (1.0)	2.1 (0.2)	3.7 (0.9)	3.9 (0.5)
Obsessive-compulsive	2.7 (0.5)	2.6 (0.3)	1.9 (0.7)	3.1 (0.4)	2.1 (0.8)	1.9 (0.4)
Drug abuse/dependence	5.2 (0.8)	6.0 (0.6)	8.2 (1.4)	5.4 (0.5)	4.5 (1.3)	5.8 (0.5)
Anorexia nervosa	0.0 (0.0)	0.1 (0.0)	0.0 (0.0)	0.1 (0.1)	0.2 (0.2)	0.1 (0.1)
Any of the covered diagnoses	25.1 (1.8)	30.2 (1.1)†	30.9 (3.1)	38.7 (1.0)†	25.6 (2.7)	31.9 (1.2)**

*Numbers in parentheses are SEs.
†P<.01
‡P<.001
**P<.05
Source: See Table 2–1.

TABLE 2–8. Urbanization of Area of Residence and *DSM-III* Lifetime Diagnosis (St. Louis Only)*

DISORDER	CENTRAL CITY (%) N=983	INNER SUBURB (%) N=1,267	SMALL TOWN/RURAL (%) N=740
Cognitive impairment†	2.6 (0.5)	0.7 (0.2)	0.6 (0.3)
Drug abuse/dependence‡	8.1 (1.6)	5.6 (0.8)	4.3 (0.8)
Alcohol abuse/dependence‡	19.4 (2.1)	15.9 (1.1)	14.0 (1.7)
Antisocial personality‡	5.7 (1.5)	3.1 (0.7)	2.4 (0.6)
Schizophrenia**	1.9 (0.5)	0.8 (0.3)	0.8 (0.4)
Panic	1.7 (0.5)	0.8 (0.2)	2.1 (0.6)
Dysthymia	4.9 (1.2)	4.5 (0.7)	2.7 (0.6)
Agoraphobia	4.6 (0.9)	4.3 (0.6)	3.7 (0.9)
Somatization	0.4 (0.2)	0.2 (0.1)	0.0 (0.0)
Manic episode	1.7 (0.7)	0.7 (0.3)	1.1 (0.5)
Major depressive episode	6.4 (1.0)	5.1 (0.9)	5.5 (1.0)
Anorexia nervosa	0.2 (0.2)	0.0 (0.0)	0.1 (0.1)
Simple phobia	6.6 (1.1)	7.6 (0.9)	6.3 (1.1)
Obsessive-compulsive	1.5 (0.3)	2.4 (0.5)	1.7 (0.6)
Schizophreniform disorder	0.0 (0.0)	0.3 (0.2)	0.0 (0.0)
Any of the covered diagnoses‡	33.7 (2.2)	32.2 (1.6)	27.5 (2.0)

*Numbers in parentheses are SEs.
†$P<.001$, central city v others.
‡$P<.05$, central city v small town/rural.
**$P<.05$, central city v suburbs.
¶$P<.05$, suburb v small town.
Source: See Table 2–1.

SCHIZOPHRENIA

Many schizophrenics are normal much of the time. The onset of schizophrenia may be slow and progressive, as if organically caused, or sudden, as when provoked by some specific event. Schizophrenic disorders can have many forms; aberrant thinking and feeling comprise a common strain in most. Schizophrenia has been defined and redefined many times during the history of its investigation. Today, four major forms are generally recognized. They are (1) paranoid, (2) hebephrenic, (3) catatonic, and (4) simple. The most severely disorganized personality is exhibited in type 2. The hebephrenic patient lives solely in fantasy and often develops grandiose delusions. Hallucinations may trigger fits of laughing even though he is depressed.

The type 1 schizophrenic is generally less removed from reality, but he or she may have systematic delusions leading to thoughts of persecution. The type 3 schizophrenic is also delusional, but he cannot communicate his delusions until the severe catatonia moderates. Before modern drug therapy, catatonic schizophrenics were incapable of motion, remaining rigid for long intervals.

The simple schizophrenic is one who, since childhood, became physically and emotionally withdrawn. This form, which does not involve the cognitive disturbances related to other forms, is less easily detected.

Mental health authorities estimate that about 1% of the population is schizophrenic. This proportion remains fairly constant even though many schizophrenics remain single and celibate. International comparative studies show that more schizophrenics are found in industrialized societies than in agrarian cultures, and in cities than in rural areas. This was also the finding in the NIMH ECA study. The 6-month prevalence of schizophrenia in men and women at each of three sites is presented in Table 2–9. The total prevalence for men and women is 0.07% and 1.6% respectively. The total of these two percentages is 1.3% and very close to the worldwide 1% estimate.

In the United States, an estimated 15.4% of all men diagnosed as suffering from mental disease are schizophrenics, whereas 18.6% of mentally ill women are schizophrenic. As expected, NIMH data show that a far greater proportion of treated mental patients are schizophrenics at a reported 36% (includes additions) as of 1979 (Table 2–10).

Various studies show a genetic link in the incidence of schizophrenia. When both parents are schizophrenic, they have a two in three chance of producing schizophrenic children. Studies of identical twins show a high correlation between schizophrenia in both members of the twin pair. The familial link suggests that schizophrenia may be continued by recessive gene carriers in the families of a schizophrenic even if he or she remains childless. Investigators have even noted that the normal female siblings of schizophrenics have more children than the general-population average. The association of schizophrenia in identical twins when the trait is known originally in one is slightly higher than 75%. In nonidentical pairs it is 15%.

TABLE 2–9. Six-Month Prevalence of DIS/*DSM-III* Schizophrenia or Schizophreniform Disorder by Sex and Age*

| | MEN | | | | | WOMEN | | | | | |
| | Age Group (in years) | | | | | Age Group (in years) | | | | | |
SITE	18–24	25–44	45–64	65+	Total Men	18–24	25–44	45–64	65+	Total Women	Total
New Haven, Conn. (%)	2.1	0.6	0.3	0.0	0.7	1.6	2.6	0.7	0.9	1.6	1.1
Baltimore (%)	1.3	0.7	0.8	0.0	0.7	1.0	3.2	0.9	0.2	1.6	1.2
St. Louis (%)	0.6	1.5	0.8	0.0	0.9	0.5	0.5	0.2	0.0	0.4	0.6

*DIS, Diagnostic Interview Schedule.
Source: Myers JK, Weissman MM, Tischler GL et al: Six-month prevalence of psychiatric disorders in three communities. *Arch Gen Psychiatr* 41: (10) 1984.

TABLE 2–10. Percent Distribution and Rate per 100,000 Civilian Population* of Additions to State and County Mental Hospitals, by Diagnosis and Age: United States, 1969, 1974, and 1979

DIAGNOSIS† AND AGE‡	1969	1974	1979	1969	1974	1979	1969	1974	1979
	Number			Percentage distribution			Rate		
Schizophrenia, total	137,007	139,832	136,870	29.9	32.2	36.0	69.2	66.4	61.7
Less than 18	4,948	3,558	3,086	1.1	0.8	0.8	7.1	5.2	4.8
18–44	94,735	98,744	104,310	20.6	22.7	27.4	139.8	128.0	118.3
45–64	34,384	33,351	26,126	7.5	7.7	6.9	83.8	77.0	59.0
65+	2,940	4,179	3,348	0.6	1.0	0.9	15.1	19.2	13.5

Sources: *National Institute of Mental Health.* Unpublished data from the Survey and Reports Branch, Division of Biometry and Epidemiology, (1969, 1974, 1979).
Notes: The data in this table, which are provided by the state agencies of mental health through the *Annual Census of Patient Characteristics, State and County Mental Hospital Inpatient Services, Additions and Resident Patients,* are reported for the fiscal year used by the particular state. For most states, it is the year ending June 30. These data will differ slightly from numbers of inpatient additions shown in Table 2–7. The latter are based on responses to the *Inventory of Mental Health Facilities* by individual state and county mental hospitals, which are given the option to report on either a calendar- or fiscal-year basis. Information on the "state" hospital in Puerto Rico is excluded.
*The populations used in the calculations of these rates are estimates of the U.S. civilian populations (provided by the Bureau of the Census and published in Series P-25 publications) as of July 1 for each respective year.
†*Diagnostic Classification* The diagnostic classification can be found in *Diagnostic and Statistical Manual of Mental Disorders* (Second Edition), American Psychiatric Association, 1968.
‡*Age* additions during year; age is reported as of the last birthday at end of reported year.

Some schizophrenics recover spontaneously. Others report cures after nutritional therapy (deficiency of vitamins B12 and B6 are said to be associated with this mental disease). The standard treatment is administration of phenothiazine drugs, such as chlorpromazine.

AUTISM

Autism is a childhood disorder similar to schizophrenia in that victims typically fail to relate to the external world. Often unresponsive and emotionally unattached—even to their parents, they prefer to be alone. Some of them exhibit a rocking motion or a tendency to repeatedly bang their heads against a wall or some other object.

At one time, parents—particularly the mother—of an autistic child—was considered to be the cause of the syndrome. It was theorized that she was cold and detached in her dealings with the child. This view has been discredited for a long time. Today, autistic children are viewed more as a puzzle of brain malfunction. One line of investigation supports the view that the brain's dopamine system may be overactive. Dopamine is a brain neurotransmitter. Drugs, such as haloperidol and the phenothiazines that inhibit dopamine, are occasionally therapeutic. Genes are also suspected of playing a role, since the families of autistic children seem to have a higher prevalence of depression, language difficulties, psychological disturbances, and anxiety. Other researchers have found that administration of triiodothyronine, a thyroid-elaborated hormone improves the condition. Marked swings from hypothyroid to hyperthyroid level in a few days have led investigators to explore how thyroid hormones affect the metabolism of brain neurotransmitters.

DEPRESSION (AFFECTIVE DISORDERS)

Depression is defined as melancholy or sadness. As with any emotion, sadness and depression can be a completely normal and reasonable response to one's experience or environment, or both. The paradigm case in which one would expect to feel sad is at the death of a loved one. But clearly many other misfortunes and losses normally elicit sorrow. This type of expected response is often referred to as an *exogenous depression* because its cause is some stimuli or situation external to the person.

Normal depression is self-limiting; it dissipates in time, often within days or months. If the sadness persists beyond a reasonable interval to the chronic state, the depression is more accurately characterized as a mental disorder. Depending on the depressive symptoms, abnormal depression can be a neurosis or, more severely, a psychosis.

Psychotic depression can exhibit either a unipolar or bipolar pattern. In the former, one is in a fairly constant depressed state. The bipolar pattern is one of mood swings from severe depression to euphoric mania and exhilaration. The latter syndrome is called *manic depression* and is regarded as a psychosis. The prevalence of affective disorders in the general population during 6 months is shown in Table 2–11.

Patients diagnosed as depressive in state and county mental hospitals totalled 8.5 million in 1979. The proportion of publicly hospitalized depressive patients was around 6% (Table 2–12).

CAUSES

The causes of depression can be either physiologic or psychological. Organically caused depression may result from hormonal or chemical imbalances and even from some well-known physical diseases, such as infectious mononucleosis, hepatitis, and atherosclerosis. Postpartum depression, after the delivery of a baby, is a common depression syndrome. It is thought to have a predominantly

TABLE 2–11. Six-Month Prevalence of DIS/*DSM-III* Affective Disorders by Sex and Age*

SITE	MEN Age Group (in years)				Total Men	WOMEN Age Group (in years)				Total Women	Total
	18–24	25–44	45–64	65+		18–24	25–44	45–64	65+		
Major depressive episode without bereavement (%)											
New Haven, Conn.	3.9	2.7	1.4	0.5	2.2	6.1	7.4	2.2	1.6	4.6	3.5
Baltimore	1.1	1.6	1.5	0.3	1.3	3.0	4.5	2.4	1.3	3.0	2.2
St. Louis	1.1	2.8	1.3	0.1	1.7	5.2	5.2	4.9	1.0	4.5	3.2
Bereavement (%)†											
New Haven	0.0	0.0	0.1	0.0	0.0	0.3	0.3	0.4	1.7	0.6	0.3
Baltimore	0.0	0.0	0.3	0.6	0.2	0.3	0.1	0.2	0.6	0.3	0.2
St. Louis	0.0	0.2	0.0	0.0	0.1	0.0	0.1	0.0	0.6	0.2	0.1
Major episode (%)											
New Haven	1.3	1.0	0.0	0.0	0.6	2.0	1.2	0.6	0.0	0.9	0.8
Baltimore	0.0	1.1	0.0	0.0	0.4	0.3	0.7	0.3	0.0	0.4	0.4
St. Louis	1.4	0.7	0.8	0.0	0.8	1.4	1.0	0.1	0.0	0.6	0.7
Dysthymia (%)‡											
New Haven	3.0	3.0	2.1	1.8	2.6	2.3	5.1	3.0	3.1	3.7	3.2
Baltimore	0.4	1.3	1.8	0.6	1.2	1.0	4.3	3.5	1.3	2.9	2.1
St. Louis	2.2	2.7	1.8	0.5	2.1	3.6	6.0	8.0	1.6	5.4	3.8
Any affective disorder (%)**											
New Haven	7.5	5.4	3.0	2.2	4.6	9.1	11.4	5.6	5.0	8.2	6.5
Baltimore	1.5	3.7	3.1	1.2	2.7	4.5	8.9	6.3	3.1	6.0	4.6
St. Louis	3.9	5.1	3.2	0.5	3.8	7.7	9.9	9.6	3.1	8.3	6.2

*DIS, Diagnostic Interview Schedule.
†Respondents meeting criteria for major depressive episode, but explaining it as bereavement.
‡DIS 2 and 3 do not have recency probes for dysthymia, so these are lifetime figures.
**Includes dysthymia.
Source: Myers JK, Weissman MM, Tischler GL et al: Six-month prevalence of psychiatric disorders in three communities. *Arch Gen Psychiat* 41: (10) 1984.

TABLE 2–12. Percentage Distribution and Rate per 100,000 Civilian Population* of Resident Patients in State and County Mental Hospitals at End of Year, by Diagnosis and Age: United States, 1969, 1974, and 1979

DIAGNOSIS† AND AGE‡	1969	1974	1979	1969	1974	1979	1969	1974	1979
		Number		Percentage distribution			Rate		
Affective (formerly depression), total	23,688	12,803	8,592	6.4	5.9	6.2	11.9	6.0	3.9
Less than 18	234	237	276	0.1	0.1	0.2	0.3	0.3	0.4
18–44	3,544	4,034	2,967	1.0	1.9	2.1	5.2	5.2	3.3
45–64	10,103	4,461	2,491	2.7	2.1	1.8	24.4	10.3	5.6
65+	9,807	4,071	2,858	2.7	1.9	2.0	49.8	18.5	11.4

Sources: *National Institute of Mental Health.* Unpublished data from the Survey and Reports Branch, Division of Biometry and Epidemiology (1969, 1974, 1979).

Notes: The data in this table, which are provided by the state agencies of mental health through the *Annual Census of Patient Characteristics, State and County Mental Hospital Inpatient Services, Additions and Resident Patients,* are reported for the fiscal year used by the particular state. For most states, it is the year ending June 30. These data will differ slightly from numbers of inpatient additions shown in Table 2–3 that are based on responses to the *Inventory of Mental Health Facilities* by individual state and county mental hospitals, which are given the option to report on either a calendar- or fiscal-year basis. Information on the "state" hospital in Puerto Rico is excluded.

*The populations used in the calculations of these rates were obtained by averaging populations (provided by the Bureau of the Census and published in Series P-25 publications) for successive years as of July 1. For example, the population for 1979 was obtained by averaging the civilian populations as of July 1, 1978 and July 1, 1979.

†*Diagnostic Classification* The diagnostic classification can be found in *Diagnostic and Statistical Manual of Mental Disorders* (Second Edition), American Psychiatric Association, 1968. The codes corresponding to the diagnostic categories shown in the tables are as follows:

Diagnostic Groupings   Diagnostic Code
Affective (formerly depression)   296, 298.0, 300.4

‡Age additions during year; age is reported as of the last birthday before addition.
**Number in 1,000s.

physiologic cause related to the change of hormone levels and relationships that occur when the body adjusts from a pregnant to a nonpregnant state. Most of the time, postpartum depression is temporary and lasts only a few days or weeks. But a low percentage of women experience a severe depression of several months that can require treatment.

Physically or organically caused depression should not be confused with depression concomitant with an illness. The latter is generally a normal reaction to not feeling well or healthy. Depression caused by the diseases mentioned above is an intrinsically caused mental disorder resulting from a person's changed biochemical condition. In contrast, depression that results from appreciating the fact that one is sick is exogenously caused and not a mental disorder but simply a reaction to misfortune.

UNIPOLAR AND BIPOLAR DEPRESSION

Recent epidemiologic research on the profile of unipolar and bipolar depression in several European countries where populations are less mobile than in the United States have led researchers to the conclusion that these two psychotic forms of depression are cyclical in 80% of the cases. These findings suggest a link between these disorders and a lack of synchrony among one's biologic rhythms or between them and the circadian cycle. The age at onset is also a predictor of disease episode frequency (Figure 2–1). The younger one is at disease onset, the fewer repeat episodes develop and the longer the well interval between periods of unipolar and bipolar disease.

The probability of relapse within 24 hours of an initial episode in the young is only 20%. In patients who are age 60 years and older at the time of their first episode, the unipolar relapse rate increases to about 70%. Among bipolar or manic-depressive patients, the

FIG. 2–1. Probability of a relapse within 24 months following the initial episode

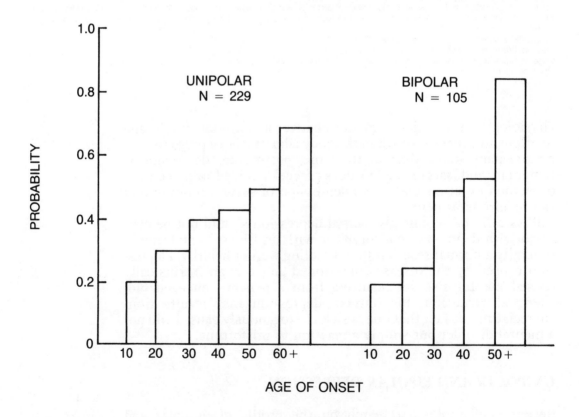

AGE OF ONSET

Source: Reprint *National Institutes of Mental Health Science* Report 1, DHEW No. ADM 79-889

probability is 85%.[1] Figure 2–1 shows the relapse probability at different ages of onset.

Researchers also find evidence of a possible genetic susceptibility in sufferers of severe depressive disorders.[2] This supposition in no way conflicts with cyclicality research dealing with depressive patients. Those who are manic depressive usually have a family history of mania; the onset of bipolar depression often occurs when they are in their third decade. Unipolar depression starts more often when people are in their fifth decade and a family history of depression is evident.

SYMPTOMS

Depression symptoms include chronic sadness, a feeling of worthlessness, low self-esteem, pessimism or hopelessness, listlessness, and lack of energy or interest in one's work. Seriously depressed people often suffer from insomnia, a decreased interest in sex or pleasure-giving activities, and a deceleration of their mental processes as reflected by broken thought patterns and slowed speech. Depressed persons are often bored. They may be irritable, forgetful, indecisive, and slow reacting. Physically, depressed people may experience loss of appetite and feel they have several physical ailments much like a hypochondriac.

Depression is the most common mental syndrome in the United States, affecting as much as 20% of the adult population. It has been referred to as the mental illness of the 1970s. During that decade, the NIMH estimated that between 4 and 8 million Americans were so severely depressed that they were unable to function. Seventy-five thousand are thought to suffer from depression psychosis, while 10 to 15 million are judged to be mildly depressed.

In 1975, a sample of randomly chosen persons was given a depression symptomatology test as an addendum to the government sponsored General Wellbeing Questionnaire. Results indicated that about 18.5 million, or 17.3% of people age 25 to 74 years had significant depression symptoms. Those questioned did not represent either institutionalized populations or the military but rather the general functioning population. Health data were also collected at the same time since the effort was incorporated into Phase 1 of the Hanes Nutrition Study.

---

[1]Grof P, Zis AP, Goodwin FK et al: "Patterns of recurrence in bipolar affective illness." Presented at the Annual Meeting of the American Psychiatric Association, 1978.
[2]Goodwin FK: Diagnosis of affective disorders. In Jarvik ME (ed): *Psychopharmacology in the Practice of Medicine.* New York: Appleton-Century Crofts, pp. 219-227, 1977.

Investigators caution that the results only indicate reports of depressive symptoms and not necessarily the prevalence of clinical depressive mental disorder. Many of the reports may reflect the prevalence of transient normal depression reactions in the population. But the latter are still worthy of study, since death and morbidity associated with depression can result from acute episodes of normal depressive reaction as well as from a chronic depressive disorder.

Answers to questions about mood and outlook were given ratings. Total ratings were scaled as indicative of the degree of depressive symptoms that a person was experiencing. Higher ratings corresponded to more severe depression.

In general, as would be expected in a U.S. population that values material gain more highly than other achievements or spiritual values and where most service and helping interractions are based on monetary exchange, those at low income levels had higher-than-average depression ratings when compared to others of their age and sex in the remaining population. The data showed that women reported more depressive symptomatology than men. With a rating or total scaled score of 7.1, men had an average depression response rate lower than that for the general population (8.7) whereas women with an average score of 10.0 had a higher-than-average rating. The standard error of the average score for the general population was 0.18. In all likelihood, then, these values for men and women are not caused by chance variation. Rather, they represent a true difference between the men and women sampled.

Women are usually cited as having a greater incidence than men of several mental diseases, including depression. Investigators caution, however, that these findings may reflect merely a greater willingness by women to seek help when they are disturbed. Analysts suspect that the large number of male alcoholics may include many with serious mental problems who have not sought professional help but who have found solace in alcohol. Still other sociologists and psychologists believe that if women have a higher rate of depression and other mental disease than men, they are simply reacting in a normal way to their cultrual role as second-class citizens. This is particularly true in cultures where women have for centuries lacked individual identity, independence, self-development, and power. None of the differences in ratings for people of various ages was statistically significant.

The largest difference for demographic cohorts was between blacks and other non-Caucasians. Blacks reported the greatest level of depression, whereas those in the "other" racial category reported the least. The greater depressive response of blacks was not distinguished statistically from the greater depressed response of those at lower income levels. Thus, the finding for people in these two categories may well be the same response. Blacks may be depressed not as a racial group but rather as a low-income group.

Those formerly married and those never married had a higher depression rating than those currently married, at 11.3 and 9.6 respectively compared with an 8.0 rating. Those in households of two or four were most happy, whereas those in households of one or seven to 15 or more were least happy. Those who either were unable to work or had never worked reported more depression. Men and women professionals were also less depressed than those in other occupations.

As already mentioned, the patterns in these data need further investigation. No conclusions can be drawn about which variable among several affecting a given group accounts primarily for their higher depression responses. Having a low income, being divorced, and being a woman all correlate with a higher-than-average depression rating in this survey. The researchers did not attempt to sort out the effects of each variable independently. This can usually be done, however, by modern statistical analysis.

Neither can it be assumed that those with higher depression ratings are abnormally or endogenously depressed. Nevertheless, depression is depression and the characteristics of normal, transient acute, or chronic situational depression can lead to or simulate depression syndromes that are considered to be abnormal, such as depressive neuroses and psychoses.

SUICIDE

Aside from impairment of daily function, exogenous depression, depressive neuroses, and to a greater extent depressive psychosis are dangerous because of the marked tendency for those who are depressed to take their own lives. Although it is true that many depressed persons never think of committing suicide and that not every suicide occurs in a depressed person, the two often go hand in hand. An estimated 75% of all suicides are the result of depression.

Table 2–13 presents data reflecting the trend in the suicide rate from 1960 to 1980 in the United States by sex and the method used. The annual number of suicides by the end of the 1970s hovered around 26,000. The number of male and female suicides that were committed in 1980 was lower than the 1977 peaks. Men resorted to firearms much more than women; the latter more commonly took poison. The data also makes clear that men commit suicide more often than women. But this does not mean that they attempt it more often. Part of the difference between the sexes may be that

TABLE 2–13. Suicides, by Sex and Method Used: 1960–1980. [Beginning 1970 excludes deaths of nonresidents of the United States. Beginning 1979 deaths classified according to the ninth revision of the *International Classification of Diseases*. For earlier years classified according to the revision in use at the time, see text, p. 61. See also *Historical Statistics, Colonial Times to 1970*, series H 979–986]

METHOD	MALE							FEMALE						
	1960	1970	1975	1977	1978	1979	1980	1960	1970	1975	1977	1978	1979	1980
Total	14,539	16,629	19,622	21,109	20,188	20,256	20,505	4,502	6,851	7,441	7,572	7,106	6,950	6,364
Firearms*	7,879	9,704	12,185	13,342	12,830	12,919	12,937	1,138	2,068	2,688	2,742	2,557	2,639	2,459
Percent of total	54.2	58.4	62.1	63.2	63.6	63.8	63.1	25.3	30.2	36.1	36.2	36.0	38.0	38.6
Poisoning†	2,631	3,299	3,297	3,340	3,105	2,974	2,997	1,699	3,285	3,129	3,147	2,912	2,754	2,456
Hanging and strangulation‡	2,576	2,422	2,815	2,982	2,759	2,783	2,997	790	831	846	848	753	742	694
Other**	1,453	1,204	1,325	1,445	1,494	1,580	1,574	875	667	778	835	884	815	755

*Includes explosives through 1978.
†Includes solids, liquids, and gases.
‡Includes suffocation.
**Beginning 1979 includes explosives.
Source: *Statistical Abstracts of the United States, 1984*

men are more successful than women when they attempt suicide.

The distribution of known suicides among men and women of different race and age is presented in Table 2–14. Overall, the U.S. suicide rate has been constant between 1950 and 1980, although the rates of several groups have reflected drastic changes. The most striking pattern change is the sharp decline in the suicide rate for older whites, particularly those in advanced age brackets older than age 55 years. Men age 55 to 64 years show a decline from 45.9 per 100,000 in 1950 to 25.8 in 1980. In the same period, the suicide rate for women in this same age group dropped from 10.7 to 9.1. The drop for white women at older ages was larger.

This is especially interesting in light of the fact that psychiatrists often refer to the melancholy that seems to attend old age, particularly in women between ages 45 and 55 years and in men ages 50 to 60. The emptying of the nest, retirement from work, and the growing awareness of one's mortality, combined sometimes with physical ailments, are typical triggers for depression. Yet the results of the 1975 depression survey did not show that older people were more depressed than younger people. Indeed, the change in older age suicide rates fly in the face of what might have been expected.

Equally startling, however, is the change that occurred among the youngest portion of the white population. Young people and adults between ages 15 and 34 years have shown a sharp rise in suicide rate. The rate among 15- to 24-year-old white males has almost doubled, whereas the rate for females in this age group has risen 40%.

These percentage increases for the young are almost the same as the percentage decreases for older adults. However, this rate reversal in the white population is not as pronounced in the black population. A look at the black population readily shows the same upward trend among black men. But the rate for black women has been relatively constant since 1950 and throughout the adult age spectrum. Only black women between age 25 and 44 years seem to have a slightly higher rate than women younger and older. A quick look at the data also shows that blacks, male and female, commit suicide much less often than whites.

These data pose several intriguing questions, especially when one reflects on renowned sociologist Émile Durkheim's social isolation explanation of suicide and a few of the societal changes that have occurred among the young and the old in the past 30 years. The most obvious change is that old and elderly adults live much more independently in 1980 than they did in 1950. Older Americans are generally much healthier than their 1950s counterparts and more financially secure because of social programs

TABLE 2–14. Death Rates for Suicide, According to Race, Sex, and Age: United States, selected years 1950–82 (data are based on the National Vital Statistics System)

RACE, SEX, AND AGE	YEAR							
	1950*	1960*	1970	1975	1979	1980	1981†	1982†
Total‡	Deaths per 100,000 resident population							
All ages, age adjusted**	11.0	10.6	11.8	12.5	11.7	11.4	11.3	11.5
All ages, crude	11.4	10.6	11.6	12.6	12.1	11.9	11.8	12.0
Under 1 year	—	—	—	—	—	—	—	—
1–4 years	—	—	—	—	—	—	—	—
5–14 years	0.2	0.3	0.3	0.4	0.4	0.4	0.4	0.3
15–24 years	4.5	5.2	8.8	11.7	12.4	12.3	12.5	12.5
25–34 years	9.1	10.0	14.1	16.1	16.3	16.0	16.2	15.5
35–44 years	14.3	14.2	16.9	17.4	15.4	15.4	14.7	16.5
45–54 years	20.9	20.7	20.0	20.1	16.5	15.9	15.9	15.9
55–64 years	27.0	23.7	21.4	19.8	16.6	15.9	14.6	15.9
65–74 years	29.3	23.0	20.8	19.6	17.8	16.9	16.9	16.7
75–84 years	31.1	27.9	21.2	19.7	20.8	19.1	18.8	19.7
85 years and over	28.8	26.0	20.4	18.6	17.9	19.2	20.7	17.2
White male								
All ages, age adjusted**	18.1	17.5	18.2	19.6	18.6	18.9	—	—
All ages, crude	19.0	17.6	18.0	19.9	19.6	19.9	—	—
Under 1 year	—	—	—	—	—	—	—	—
1–4 years	—	—	—	—	—	—	—	—
5–14 years	0.3	0.5	0.5	0.8	0.6	0.7	—	—
15–24 years	6.6	8.6	13.9	19.3	20.5	21.4	—	—
25–34 years	13.8	14.9	19.9	24.0	25.4	25.6	—	—
35–44 years	22.4	21.9	23.3	24.4	22.4	23.5	—	—
45–54 years	34.1	33.7	29.5	29.7	24.0	24.2	—	—
55–64 years	45.9	40.2	35.0	31.9	26.3	25.8	—	—
65–74 years	53.2	42.0	38.7	36.0	33.4	32.5	—	—
75–84 years	61.9	55.7	45.5	43.2	48.0	45.5	—	—
85 years and over	61.9	61.3	50.3	51.1	50.2	52.8	—	—
White female								
All ages, age adjusted**	5.3	5.3	7.2	7.3	6.3	5.7	—	—
All ages, crude	5.5	5.3	7.1	7.3	6.5	5.9	—	—
Under 1 year	—	—	—	—	—	—	—	—
1–4 years	—	—	—	—	—	—	—	—
5–14 years	0.1	*0.1	0.1	0.2	0.3	0.2	—	—
15–24 years	2.7	2.3	4.2	4.9	4.9	4.6	—	—
25–34 years	5.2	5.8	9.0	8.8	7.8	7.5	—	—
35–44 years	8.2	8.1	13.0	12.6	10.1	9.1	—	—
45–54 years	10.5	10.9	13.5	13.8	11.6	10.2	—	—

55–64 years	10.7	10.9	12.3	11.5	9.9	9.1
65–74 years	10.6	8.8	9.6	9.4	7.8	7.0
75–84 years	8.4	9.2	7.2	7.5	6.7	5.7
85 years and over	8.9	6.1	6.1	4.8	5.0	5.8
Black male						
All ages, age adjusted**	7.0	7.8	9.9	11.4	12.5	11.4
All ages, crude	6.3	6.4	8.0	9.9	11.5	10.3
Under 1 year	—	—	—	—	—	—
1–4 years	—	—	—	—	—	—
5–14 years	*0.1	*0.1	*0.1	0.1	0.2	0.3
15–24 years	4.9	4.1	10.5	12.7	14.0	12.3
25–34 years	9.3	12.4	19.2	23.4	24.9	21.8
35–44 years	10.4	12.8	12.6	16.0	16.9	15.6
45–54 years	10.4	10.8	13.8	12.4	13.8	12.0
55–64 years	16.5	16.2	10.6	10.7	12.8	11.7
65–74 years	10.0	11.3	8.7	11.6	13.5	11.1
75–84 years	—	*6.6	*8.9	11.7	10.5	10.5
85 years and over	6.2	*6.9	10.3	4.3	15.4	18.9
Black female						
All ages, age adjusted**	1.7	1.9	2.9	2.9	2.9	2.4
All ages, crude	1.5	1.6	2.6	2.7	2.8	2.2
Under 1 year	—	—	—	—	—	—
1–4 years	—	—	—	—	—	—
5–14 years	—	*0.0	*0.2	*0.1	0.1	0.1
15–24 years	1.8	1.3	3.8	3.2	3.3	2.3
25–34 years	2.6	3.0	5.7	5.4	5.4	4.1
35–44 years	2.0	3.0	3.7	4.0	4.1	4.6
45–54 years	3.5	3.1	3.7	4.0	2.9	2.8
55–64 years	1.1	*3.0	*2.0	3.4	3.8	2.3
65–74 years	1.9	*2.3	*2.9	3.0	2.6	1.7
75–84 years	2.4	*1.3	*1.7	1.2	2.5	1.4
85 years and over	—	—	3.2	—	1.0	—

*Includes deaths of nonresidents of the United States.

†Provisional data.

‡Includes all races and both sexes.

**Age adjusted by the direct method to the total population of the United States as enumerated in 1940, using 11 age groups.

Note: For the data years shown, the code numbers for suicide are based on the then current International Classification of Diseases; for 1950, the Sixth Revision, Nos. E963, E970–E979; for 1960, the Seventh Revision, Nos. E963, E970–E979; for 1970–78, the Eighth Revision, Adapted for Use in the United States, Nos. E950–E959; and for 1979–82, the Ninth Revision, Nos. E950–E959.

Sources: National Center for Health Statistics: *Vital Statistics of the United States*, Vol. 11, 1950–80. Public Health Service. Washington. U.S. Government Printing Office; Annual summary of births, deaths, marriages, and divorces, United States, 1982. *Monthly Vital Statistics Report.* Vol. 31–No. 13. DHHS Pub. No. (PHS) 83–1120. Public Health Service. Hyattsville, Md., Sept. 27, 1983; Data computed by the Division of Analysis from data compiled by the Division of Vital Statistics; U.S. Bureau of the Census: Population estimates and projections. *Current Population Reports.* Series P-25, No. 310. Washington. U.S. Government Printing Office, June 1965; *1950 Nonwhite Population by Race*, Special Report P-E, No. 38. Washington. U.S. Government Printing Office, 1951; General population characteristics, United States summary, 1960 and 1970. *U.S. Census of Population.* Final reports PC(1)-1B and PC(1)-B1. Washington, U.S. Government Printing Office, 1961 and 1972.

introduced during the 1930s (Social Security, e.g.) This greater economic and physical strength has also enabled older adults to live in separate housing, often hundreds of miles away from their adult children, instead of with their children in an extended family as was common in the past.

Concurrently, loss of the extended family has put much more strain on the young nuclear family, consisting of two married adults and their children. Young adults must deal with the challenges of economic development and child rearing without the experience or daily support of other more experienced family members. Coincidentally, the isolation of the nuclear family becomes even greater as families fragment into smaller social units through divorce. After 1960, divorce construed as a measure of alienation was a sound predictor of suicide.[3] Increasingly, children are being raised by only one adult head of household who often cannot give them the time and attention they need. Sociologists describe these changes in social organization of the family—and indeed the disappearance of what was once considered to be a family—as *fragmentation.*

Psychiatrists who analyze increasing child and teenage suicide must also consider the hypothesis that pressure to achieve and to obtain good grades in school may be a cause of teenage stress in the United States. This hypothesis seems dubious, however, since SAT scores declined in the United States for 22 years after 1960 by a magnitude that cannot be explained solely by wider participation in such testing. This period corresponds to the trend in increasing suicide among the young. If achievement is related to pressure to achieve, then a pressure to learn and obtain good grades has been less and less prevalent since 1960. So, too, a host of pressures—such as fear of fatal infectious disease and the need to support one's parents or to work in a stultifying sweatshop—is notably lacking in today's United States.

A more insightful construction may be that youngsters have a decreased ability to deal with today's pressures, regardless of type and extent. Lack of familial and community support, which correlate with the increasing rate of teenage and young adult suicide, are likely reasons why coping mechanisms seem to fail more today than heretofore.

As was stated in a 1982 suicide report by the World Health Organization, "Currently there is some consensus for the view that attempted suicide is usually an impulsive response to an intolerable social situation. However, there are no indications that social

---

[3]World Health Organization *EURO Reports and Studies,* p 24, 1974.

problems and distress levels have increased to the same extent though some would argue that levels of tolerance to distress have fallen markedly."[3]

Another factor rarely mentioned by professionals in their public discussion of this problem is the rate of substance abuse among the young that has risen in the last 30 years. It corresponds directly to the trend of increased suicide in the same age group. Many illicitly used and abused substances have mind- and mood-altering effects. They not uncommonly lead to psychotic disorders, depression, and ultimately suicide. Turning to drugs can be a stress-related behavior. What isn't generally realized is that this behavorial response exacerbates existing coping inadequacies. Commonly, it leads to a total breakdown of all coping mechanisms. Indeed, drug use by mentally stable individuals often causes depression and psychotic disorders.

Another intriguing aspect of the data just described is that blacks—who have had a long experience with stressful living conditions, family fragmentation, violence, and substance abuse—report more depression symptoms than do whites. But blacks have a much lower suicide rate than do whites in the United States. The profile of those who attempt suicide both in the United States and Europe is one of greater prevalence among the young, women, and members of the lower socioeconomic classes. Attempts are more frequent among the divorced, alcoholics, criminals, the unemployed, and those with a history of debt and family violence. The lower rate among U.S. blacks who have for historical reasons been largely confined to lower socioeconomic levels of U.S. society seems to belie the explanation of suicide just reviewed.

The suicide rate is highest in the south and west, particularly in Nevada and New Mexico. The rate is also high in Alaska (Table 2-15). It is intriguing to note that Utah, which lies between Nevada and New Mexico, has a much lower suicide rate than either state. Utah, the home of the Mormon Church, reports lower rates of cancer and heart disease as well. Mormans have been the subject of much medical epidemiologic investigation. This group has a visible commitment to strong family and community ties and abstinence from affective substances, such as alcohol, caffeine, nicotine, and hard drugs.

Although the United States is currently focusing on the problem of suicide, especially among its young adults, the overall rate has been fairly steady for years. Additionally, the U.S. rate of 18.6% reported internationally is much lower than that for several other

---

[3]Ibid, p 32

TABLE 2–15. Deaths per 100,000 Population Enumerated as of April 1, 1980 by Place of Residence. (It excludes nonresidents of U.S. causes of death classified according to ninth revision of the *International Classification of Diseases*)

REGION, DIVISION AND STATE	SUICIDE
U.S.	11.9
Regions:	
Northeast	9.6
North Central	11.0
South	12.4
West	14.8
New England	9.5
Maine	12.5
New Hampshire	11.0
Vermont	14.7
Massachusetts	8.2
Rhode Island	11.2
Connecticut	8.9
Middle Atlantic	9.6
New York	9.5
New Jersey	7.4
Pennsylvania	11.1
E. No. Central	10.9
Ohio	11.9
Indiana	10.4
Illinois	9.3
Michigan	11.5
Wisconsin	11.7
W. No. Central	11.2
Minnesota	10.8
Iowa	11.0
Missouri	11.9
North Dakota	11.0
South Dakota	12.7
Nebraska	10.1
Kansas	10.9
South Atlantic	12.7
Delaware	11.9
Maryland	10.8
District of Columbia	9.9
Virginia	13.4
West Virginia	12.5
North Carolina	11.2
South Carolina	9.5
Georgia	12.6
Florida	15.4
E. So. Central	11.6
Kentucky	12.8
Tennessee	12.2
Alabama	11.2
Mississippi	9.2
W. So. Central	12.3
Arkansas	11.6
Louisiana	12.1
Oklahoma	13.1
Texas	12.3
Mountain	16.2

Montana	14.5
Idaho	13.1
Wyoming	16.0
Colorado	16.3
New Mexico	17.4
Arizona	16.9
Utah	13.2
Nevada	22.9
Pacific	14.3
Washington	13.3
Oregon	14.6
California	14.5
Alaska	16.9
Hawaii	11.4

*Includes allied conditions.
Source: *U.S. National Center for Health Statistics,* unpublished data.

TABLE 2–16. Deaths from Suicide in European Region of the World Health Organization (latest year available)

COUNTRY	YEAR	MALES		FEMALES		TOTAL	
		No.	Rate per 100,000 population	No.	Rate per 100,000 population	No.	Rate per 100,000 population
Austria	1980	1342	37.8	590	14.9	1932	25.7
Belgium	1977	1201	25.0	673	13.4	1874	19.1
Bulgaria	1980	842	19.1	364	8.2	1206	13.6
Czechoslovakia	1975	2345	32.5	896	11.8	3241	21.9
Denmark	1980	1039	41.1	579	22.3	1618	31.6
Finland	1978	963	41.9	237	9.7	1200	25.2
France	1978	6447	24.7	2711	10.0	9158	17.2
Germany							
Fed. Rep. of	1980	8332	28.3	4536	14.1	12808	20.9
Greece	1979	186	4.0	91	1.9	277	2.9
Hungary	1980	3344	64.5	1465	26.5	4809	44.9
Iceland	1980	14	12.2	10	8.8	24	10.5
Ireland	1978	106	6.4	57	3.5	163	4.9
Italy	1978	2563	9.3	1092	3.8	3657	6.4
Luxembourg	1980	35	19.7	12	6.5	47	12.9
Malta	1977	0	—	—	—	0	—
Netherlands	1980	901	12.8	529	7.4	1430	10.1
Norway	1980	370	18.3	137	6.6	507	12.4
Poland	1979	3766	21.8	732	4.0	4498	12.7
Portugal	1979	701	15.0	251	4.8	952	9.7
Spain	1978	1094	6.1	413	2.2	1507	4.1
Sweden	1980	1137	27.6	473	11.3	1610	19.4
Switzerland	1980	1126	36.7	493	15.2	1621	25.7
United Kingdom:							
England & Wales	1980	2629	11.0	1692	6.7	4321	8.8
Northern Ireland	1978	38	5.0	32	4.1	70	4.5
Scotland	1981	339	13.6	177	6.6	516	10.0

Source: WHO data bank.

countries, including Austria, Belgium, and Czechoslovakia (Table 2–16). The rate reported internationally for the United States at 18.6% in 1981 is higher than the age-adjusted rate of 11.5%. The difference is no doubt due to a different method of computation and a smaller base population. The higher figure is retained here for purposes of comparison with other international data.

Figure 2–2 shows the percentage change in European female suicide rates by age groups in the 1960s and 1970s. Among countries with the highest percentage increases in persons age 15 to 24 years are Ireland, Norway, and Scotland. At age 25 to 34 years, the Netherlands, Ireland and Norway again show the largest increases. Belgium joins them in the older age category (35 to 44 years). At age 75+ years, Hungary and the Federal Republic of West Germany show higher percentage increases than do most other countries. When looking at these data, the reader should remember that percentage increases can be deceiving. For example, Ireland has high percentage increases on a very low rate that is among the lowest of the 18 countries compared.

The male suicide rates for Austria, Denmark, Finland, Ireland, Luxembourg, Norway, Portugal, and Sweden have generally increased. Those for the Federal Republic of West Germany, Italy, Switzerland, England, and Wales have generally dropped. The percentage changes in the European male suicide rates in the 1960s and 1970s are graphed in Figure 2–3. In the youngest age group (15 to 24 years), Ireland and Norway again show the highest percentage gain. But other countries, such as Belgium, Finland, France, and the Netherlands also show large gains. By age 25 to 34 years, men in Belgium, Ireland, and the Netherlands lead the list. At older ages the percentage increases are generally narrower than among the young. Many European countries show substantial percentage decreases. Among them are Greece, Finland, France, Italy, Poland, England and Wales, Scotland, and Switzerland.

The European suicide data show large percentage increases for young women and men, but smaller increases in the rates of women and particularly men at older ages. In these same older categories, many countries actually showed a rate drop for women. For men, the fall was even more pronounced.

The changes in suicide rates and their variability from country to country have led researchers to study the rise and fall of suicide rates in countries when some large variable, such as war or economic depression, also affected peoples' lives. One of the sociological explanations for a high suicide rate is a lack of social cohesion. Those who cite this factor as a possible cause of suicide point to the alienation and anomie of modern industrial societies. Individuals do not have a strong sense of belonging to a social unit

FIG. 2–2. Percentage change in female suicide rates from 1960–1964 to 1975–1977 by different age groups in 18 European countries

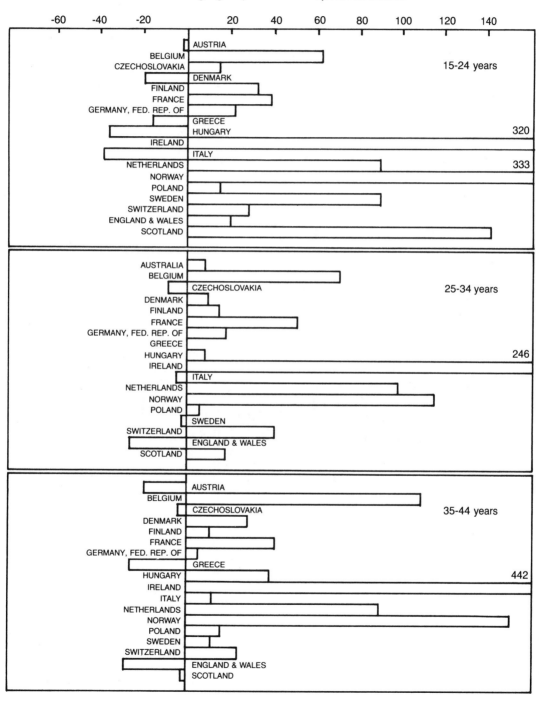

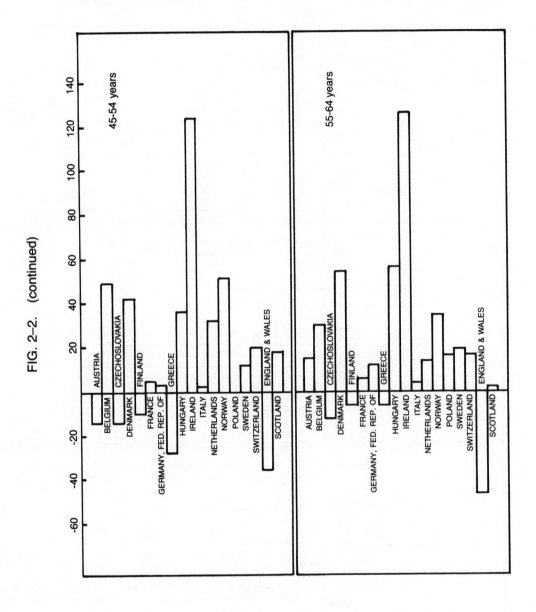

FIG. 2–2. (continued)

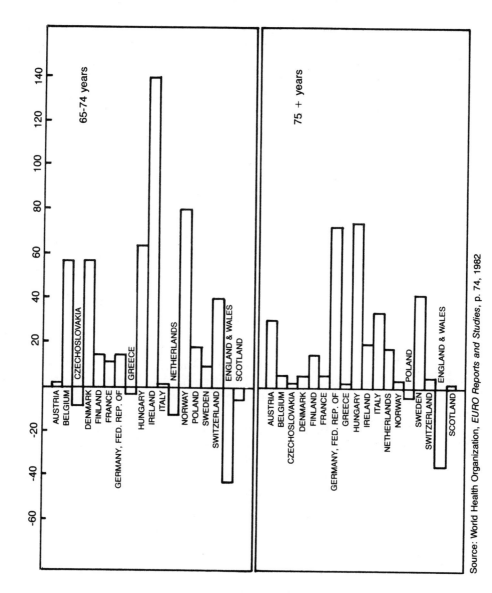

FIG. 2–2. (continued)

Source: World Health Organization, *EURO Reports and Studies*, p. 74, 1982

such as the community or family. Social relationships are fragmented; so are the activities persons engage in whereby a unified sense of self becomes a disunified collection of roles.

A test of this hypothesis can be found in the collection of suicide data for those years in which countries were at war. The premise is that the threat from an external enemy in war creates a sense of national unity, purpose, belonging, and dedication to one's national community. The percentage change in suicide rates for men and women in various European countries from 1938 to 1944 when many of these countries were participants in World War II was sizeable for many (Table 2–17).

Some of the countries constituted the battleground and involved the entire population—both soldier and civilian. Whatever the effect of the war, one would expect to see it in both men and women. Other countries were not the actual battleground but sent soldiers to the battle sites beyond their borders. The population of these countries were involved in the war differently, because the men left to fight and the women stayed behind, carrying on everyday life. Table 2–18 also shows rates for neutral countries. Interestingly, the male suicide rate for all listed countries except Spain declined, during the war, often to a large extent. The rate in Austria declined by 54%. The female rate did not decline as uniformly; where there was a decline, it was often smaller than the male decline. When Australian men had a 40% decline during this time, Australian women had a rate decline of 2%. But in New Zealand, the female rate actually increased. The rate among Danish and Norwegian women jumped 59% and 85%, respectively. But in countries like France and Italy where much of the war was fought, the suicide rates for both men and women declined significantly. (Table 2–17).

Another suspected factor in suicide is economic status, particularly if it changes suddenly. It did for many people in the Great Depression. The data vary, but the suicide rates for both sexes in most age categories increased. Suicide rates rose among middle-aged people of both sexes. Still, some of the highest percentage increases were among the young. The increase among young Finnish males is the outstanding example at 108% (Table 2–18).

Between 1961 and 1974, the hypothesis that communal and familial fragmentation in complex industrialized societies is a major cause of suicide was tested through regression analysis on data gathered for European countries. The variables chosen as measures of fragmentation and isolation were (1) the percentage of the population younger than age 15 and older than 65 years, (2) room occupancy, and (3) women in tertiary education.

A decline in the number of children, lower occupancy per room,

FIG. 2–3. Percentage change in male suicide rates from 1960-1964 to 1975–1977 by different age groups in 18 European countries

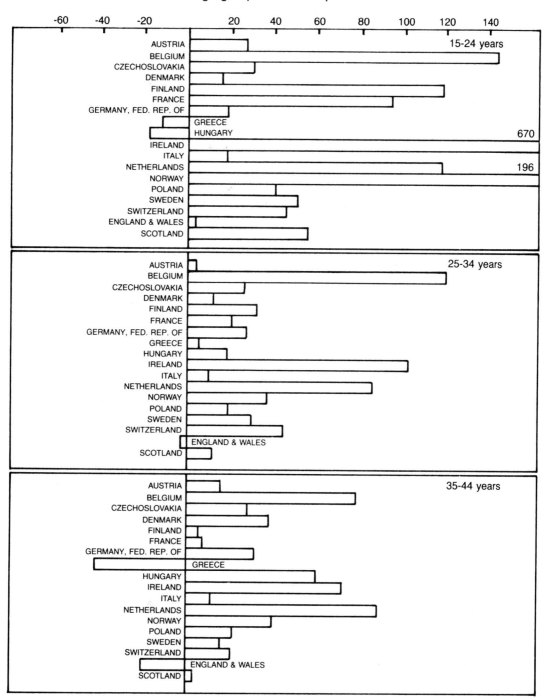

FIG. 2-3. (continued)

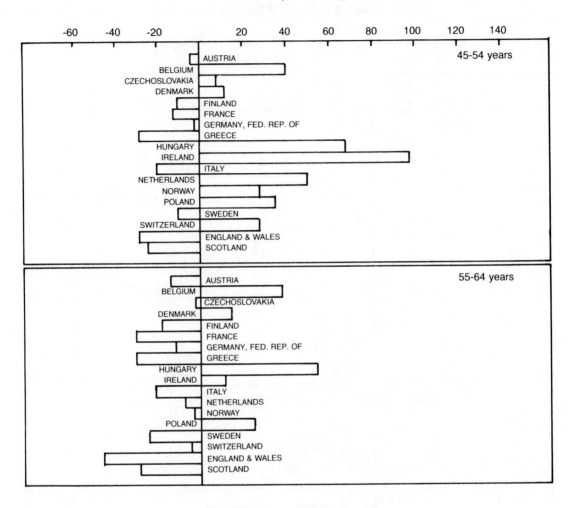

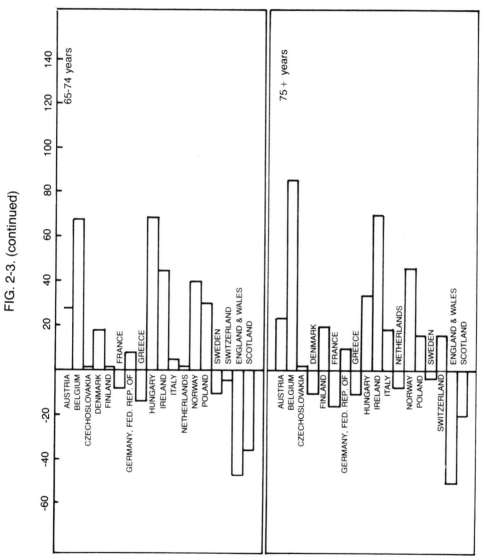

FIG. 2-3. (continued)

Source: World Health Organization, *EURO Reports and Studies*, p. 74, 1982.

and increases in the number of women in tertiary education indicated smaller family units with fewer people at home and thus less social support and cohesion for individuals. The light bars (Figure 2–4) show what researchers predicted would happen to the suicide rate based on changes in the variables selected. By comparison, the dark bars show the change in the actual rates for various European countries. For every country except France and Italy, the suicide rate changed in the same direction as predicted. Switzerland, Belgium, and Norway had a predicted increase that was greater compared to other countries than the actual increase.

TABLE 2–17. Effect of War on Suicide Rates by Sex in Belligerent and Neutral Countries (suicides per 100,000 population aged 15 years and over)

COUNTRY	MALE			FEMALE		
	1938	1944	Percentage difference	1938	1944	Percentage difference
Belligerent countries						
Australia	16.4	9.9	−40	5.0	4.9	− 2
Austria*	60.7	28.1	−54	28.6	13.8	−52
Belgium	27.6	18.1	−34	8.6	6.5	−24
Canada	13.1	8.9	−32	3.7	3.2	−14
Denmark	28.9	24.0	−17	12.9	20.5	+59
Finland	32.8	27.7	−16	7.3	5.3	−27
France	31.0	18.2	−41	8.9	6.1	−31
Italy	11.0	6.0	−45	3.6	2.0	−44
Japan†‡	21.0	18.7	−11	12.9	12.9	0
Netherlands	11.6	7.4	−36	5.4	5.6	+ 4
New Zealand	19.5	14.6	−25	5.1	5.7	+12
Norway	10.7	8.2	−23	5.3	9.8	+85
Union of South Africa	15.5	10.7	−31	5.0	3.4	−32
United Kingdom:						
England & Wales	18.0	13.5	−25	8.2	5.8	−29
Northern Ireland	6.9	5.6	−19	6.9	5.6	−19
Scotland	12.3	9.1	−26	6.3	4.5	−29
United States	23.5	14.9	−37	6.9	5.4	−22
Neutral countries						
Chile	6.8	6.5	− 4	2.5	2.3	− 8
Ireland	4.7	4.6	− 2	1.8	0.6	−67
Portugal	16.6	13.9	−16	5.0	4.8	− 4
Spain**	6.9	8.8	+28	2.3	2.6	+13
Sweden	25.0	20.6	−18	6.8	5.7	−16
Switzerland	38.4	37.2	− 3	11.6	14.7	+27

*Nearest figures available for Austria were for 1946 (1938 "Anschluss")
†Japan was also at war in 1938
‡Nearest figures available for Japan were for 1947
**Civil war in Spain in 1938
Source: World Health Organization, *EURO Reports and Studies*, p 74, 1982.

England, Greece, and Scotland were expected to show a drop in their suicide rates based on changes in the regressed variables. And all showed declines.

For both males and females, the suicide rates in England and Wales from 1900 to 1974 declined most sharply in older age groups. The rate for females age 15 to 24 years actually increased, but the increase in this group is obscured by the overall dramatic and predicted rate decline. It might be assumed from this observation that the contribution variables to suicide for both sexes in most age groups are not the major factors in young female suicides (Figure 2–5).

TABLE 2–18. Changes in the Incidence of Suicide by Sex and Age in Selected Countries between 1921–1922 and 1931–1932 (economic depression)*

COUNTRY	MALES			FEMALES		
	20–39 years	40–49 years	>60 years	20–39 years	40–49 years	>60 years
Australia	+ 25	+ 10	0	0	+ 17	− 7
Belgium	+ 29	+ 19	+19	− 6	+ 18	+ 2
Canada	+ 29	+ 48	+33	+ 32	+ 15	+23
Chile	+ 96	+150	+41	+ 90	+200	N.K.†
Denmark	+ 13	+ 22	− 9	+ 88	+ 6	+ 5
Finland	+108	+ 58	+68	+ 39	+ 42	+13
France	+ 8	+ 3	0	− 5	+ 5	− 5
Germany	− 3	+ 17	+ 1	+ 13	+ 28	+15
Italy	+ 5	+ 76	+55	− 4	+ 47	+52
Netherlands	− 14	+ 11	− 1	+ 15	+ 54	+38
New Zealand	− 10	+ 26	+19	− 5	+ 28	+47
Norway	+ 22	+ 35	+49	+ 63	+ 18	−24
Portugal	+ 14	+ 61	+54	− 10	+ 5	+46
Spain	− 5	+ 36	+23	+ 14	+ 26	+33
Sweden	− 9	+ 8	− 2	+ 3	− 2	−15
Switzerland	+ 13	+ 5	+ 5	− 4	+ 13	− 9
Union of South Africa	+ 10	− 4	+17	+ 63	+104	+35
United Kingdom:						
England and Wales	+ 41	+ 20	+16	+ 42	+ 32	+45
Scotland	+ 56	+ 77	+76	+128	+ 91	+68
United States	+ 6	+ 28	+36	+ 19	+ 21	+20
Number which increased	15	19	15	13	19	14
Number which decreased	5	1	3	6	1	5
No change, or number not known	0	0	2	1	0	1
Sign test two tailed P	0.042	<0.001	0.008	0.168	<0.001	0.064
Number of times age group had:						
greatest increase	6	11	3	5	10	5
greatest decrease	5	1	1	4	0	4

*Percentage change, mortality around 1920–1921=100.
†N.K.=not known.
Source: World Health Organization, *EURO Reports and Studies*, p 74, 1982.

FIG. 2–4. Observed and predicted changes in suicide rates in 18 European countries, 1961–1963 to 1972–1974. The results were obtained by multiple regression analysis, using percentage changes in social variables. Variables included: percentage of the population under 15 and over 65 years of age; room occupancy; women in tertiary education. Multiple R = 0.92.

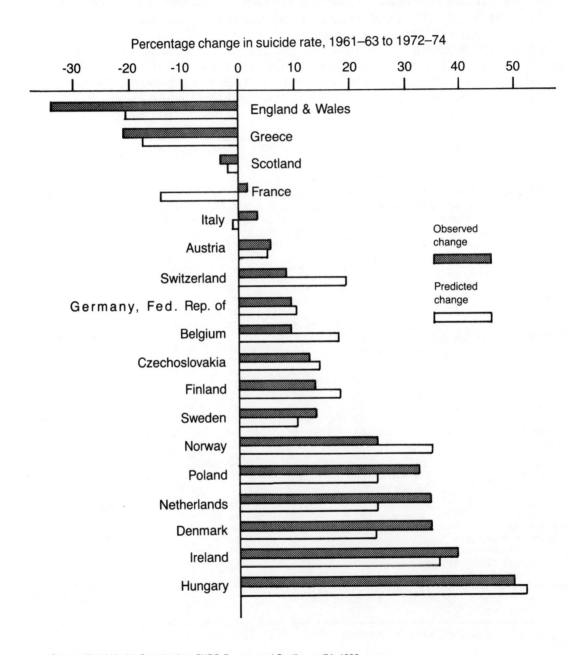

Parents, teachers, and clergymen have organized awareness, education, and support groups in an attempt to stem the rising suicide rate among the young. Many suicide hotlines have been implemented in the last 10 years to help those in acute need. This Samaritan measure was evaluated in England to see if it lowered suicide rates. When the rates in towns that had the hotlines were compared with those which did not, the rates showed little difference except that the rate in Samaritan towns actually declined less than the control town rate 5 years after the hotlines were installed.

This surprising finding may be explained by the increased societal awareness and concern generally that led to the installing of hotlines in some towns. The towns without hotlines may

FIG. 2–5. Comparison of suicide rates in control towns and Samaritan towns

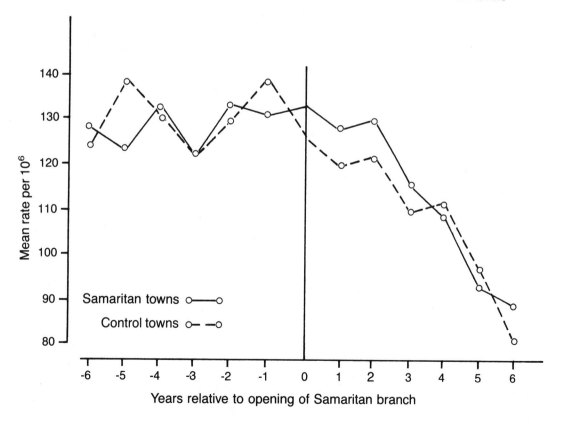

Source: World Health Organization, *EURO Reports and Studies*, p. 74, 1982.

nevertheless have had increased discussion of the problem among the general population, schools, churches, and family groups and a sensitization to those in need of emotional support.

Suicide is clearly the most serious result of depression, but substance abuse is also common. Thus, there have also been attempts to teach depressed people that escape into substance abuse only worsens the situation and that therapeutic help is available. Persons are also being counseled that some depression, including holiday and seasonal depression, is normal and predictable. One should allow oneself time to work through sadness while trying to take a positive approach to one's situation.

Researchers are finding that some depression is biological. And other avenues of study into the possible causes of inexplicable depression are also being investigated. One of them is the relationship between light and depression. People are generally more depressed in the winter when the days are shorter.

Persons with serious, lasting depression are being treated with several kinds of drugs. Tricyclic antidepressants elevate mood when used over several weeks. Severe depression is being treated with drugs known as MAO inhibitors. Both therapies require close professional monitoring since they can have undesirable side effects. They cannot be used at all if the sufferer also has certain medical conditions, such as heart or kidney disease. Lithium is another chemical agent that has worked well in controlling manic depression.

NEUROSIS

Accurately assessing the number of people suffering from neurotic disorders is difficult. But some idea of the magnitude of these disorders can be obtained from reviewing patient discharges with the diagnosis of neurosis (Table 2–19). In 1981, neurosis was one of the five leading diagnoses for men and women ages 15 to 65 years who were hospitalized. Their average length of stay was 9 days.

In 1981, the hospitalized patients diagnosed as having a neurosis totaled 1,179,000. Neurotic symptoms include tremor, dizziness, heart palpitations, shallow breathing, and extreme anxiety. Others are hysteria and obsessional behavior. Observation of hysteria patients led Freud to formulate psychoanalytic treatment principles. Modified by his successors Adler and Jung, this therapy is still used today, together with several others.

FORMS

TABLE 2–19. Hospitalization for Neurosis 1981, Days of Care and Average Length of Stay

AGE (Years)	Discharges per 1,000 persons	Rate per 1,000 persons	Days of care per 1,000 persons	Average stay (days)
		MALES		
15–44	179	3.4	36.4	10.6
45–64	55	2.6	25.4	9.8
		FEMALES		
15–44	238	4.4	38.4	8.7
45–64	85	3.7	34.3	9.4

Source: *Statistical Abstracts of the United States,* 1984

The major forms of neurotic disorder are anxiety neurosis, depersonalization, neurotic depression, hypochondriasis, hysteria, neurasthenia, obsessive compulsive neurosis, and phobia.

Anxiety neurosis occurs when one feels dread, foreboding, or fear for no apparent reason. It is sometimes described as free-floating anxiety differing from the normal pangs of fear that people develop in response to a specific dread-inducing situation or event. Age of onset is often in the second decade. Most anxiety neurotics can usually function and do not require hospitalization. Some of them eventually recover. Others respond to sedatives and mild tranquilizers, reassurance, and assertiveness training. The last-mentioned item enables them to take command of their lives.

Like anxiety, depersonalization can be either a symptom of other neuroses or a disorder itself. Those exhibiting *depersonalization*, feel insubstantial, dead, or detached from their bodies. Depersonalized young adults have a warped sense of time and a belief that the world is coming to an end. Some investigators also believe that depersonalization is a defense against an incipient psychotic reaction. Persistent episodes require therapeutic treatment.

In *hypochondriasis*, the sufferer dwells on details of body function and minor complaints, often convinced that he or she is seriously ill. These worries are a means of controlling others and getting their attention and sympathy. Developing in middle age, the condition is associated with midlife crisis. Behavior modification techniques of reconditioning and reinforcement are employed to resolve it.

Hysteria is a neurosis that takes many forms. Some of them mimic physical disabilities, such as sudden deafness, a loss of sensation, or an inability to speak. Some hysterics lose their memory. Multiple personalities have also been attributed to this disorder. About 10% of all neuroses are of this type. One form of hysteria that has received much attention lately is *anorexia nervosa*. This condition was first noted in England and France about 100 years ago. The earliest report is attributed to Richard Morton who, in 1689, described someone skeletonlike, who was suffering from a nervous consumption.

Many investigators have sought physical causes for the disorder, such as hypopituitarism. The latter can be detected by assay of pituitary tropic hormones. Today, it is believed that many anorexics suffer from emotional neurosis. The most conspicuous feature of the condition is emaciation. Anorexics refuse or fail to realize that they are too thin. Secondary symptoms are amenorrhea, intolerance to cold, low blood pressure, and slowed heart beat.

Psychologically, anorexics cannot accept the fact that they are not fat or that they are hungry. They have an inordinate fear of weight gain. Some anorexics dread failure; they strive for perfection and have a strong desire to achieve and to gain social approval. Lack of food prompts binge eating and bulimic (abnormally excessive eating) behavior in many. The fatality estimate is as high as 10% to 15%. Studies of English boarding-school girls between ages 14 to 18 years indicate an incidence of 1 in 200 in such girls. Although exact incidence information in the United States is not readily available, the disorder is common among college-age women. Female anorexics outnumber males by 9 to 1. But recent reports from England say that the incidence in males may be higher than previously thought. Treatment requires hospitalization and extensive psychotherapeutic measures.

Psychiatrists hypothesize that when hysterics simulate a physical incapacity of some sort, they are trying to avoid stress or pain. The hysteric is commonly described as being histrionic, manipulative, demanding, dishonest, unconcerned about his disability, and (usually) unaware of the depth of his egocentrism. They are believed to have been deprived of attention and love from their parents during the early years of life.

Treatment often involves hypnosis and drug therapy. Many therapists, however, also believe that uncovering the cause of the neurosis relieves the hysteria more permanently.

Sigmund Freud believed that the United States with its common frenetic pace was the ideal incubator for *neurasthenia,* or "tired nerves" as it was commonly called. This neurotic reaction is typically referred to as a nervous breakdown, resulting from overwork and stress. This neurosis is characterized by fatigue, sleepiness, lack of enthusiasm, and an inability to concentrate or complete a task. It is incriminated in 10% of all neurotic disorders. Tranquilizers and promoting understanding and self-confidence are therapeutic.

Sufferers of *obsessive compulsive neurosis* are difficult to treat. They may have many overlapping symptoms, such as an obsessive idea and a strong compulsion toward behavior directed at allaying fears promoted by obsessive thinking. The compulsive behavior can align itself with hysteria symptoms or phobic fears. The rate of reported obsessives was noted for a 6-month period according to age and sex at three research sites (Table 2–20). Psychoanalytic treatment is directed toward strengthening the patient's ego and encouraging him to identify the patterns of defense he has been using.

Other therapies include hypnosis and acting out the obsession. Others use hypnosis with a combination of agents to relieve attendant depression. Behavioral therapists believe that unlearning the compulsive behavior works best. Punishment meted out by the therapist and the patient together is effective in eliminating compulsive behavior as are small rewards given at intervals. The patient may be asked to perform his compulsive tasks to the point of exhaustion. This satiation therapy teaches the patient that performance of the compulsive behavior, even a facial twitch, is under his own control.

Phobia is included under the umbrella of panic disorders by some researchers. As its name, derived from Greek, suggests, a phobia is an overall pattern of fear and avoidance. Fear is usually an entirely normal reaction to one's circumstance. But when a fear dominates one's life or is blown out of all proportion to the actual danger posed, it then constitutes a phobic neurosis. Nonstatistical observation estimates that 10 million Americans suffer from phobic neuroses. Data collected by the NIMH indicates that the 6-month prevalence rate for men varies between 0.9% and 8.6%, whereas the rate for women varies from site to site, between 1.2% and 13.4% (Table 2–21). In the last decade, NIMH-funded phobia clinics have emerged. The one at New York's Long Island Jewish-Hillside Medical Center in New Hyde Park uses behavior therapy techniques and reports a cure rate of 80%.

The most serious phobia noted today is the fear of leaving one's own home. Some psychotherapists working with agoraphobics believe that as many as 6 persons of every 1,000 suffer from this disorder. Four of 5 of them are thought to be women. Patients are treated by desensitization techniques in which they gradually venture out to a store or some other public place, perhaps going no farther than the mailbox on the first outing. Many patients are also given imipramine. This is an antidepressant that prevents the panic that typically attends anxiety. Investigators report a 91% success rate.

PERSONALITY DISORDERS

The prevalence of some personality disorders in the general, noninstitutionalized population in St. Louis when studied by the NIMH varied from 2.1% in men to 0.5% in women (Table 2–22).

The major personality disorders: paranoid, schizoid, passive-aggressive, and sociopathic-psychopathic are represented in the institutionalized population at the rate of 1.5 per 100,000 population as of 1979 (Table 2–23).

The paranoid personality becomes manifest after age 30 years. Characteristically, it involves delusions of reference, of influence, or of grandeur, persecution, and morbid jealousy. More common among women, it is often treated by outpatient psychotherapy and

TABLE 2–20. Six-Month Prevalence of DIS/*DSM-III* Panic and Obsessive-Compulsive Disorders by Sex and Age*

| | MEN | | | | | WOMEN | | | | | |
| | Age Group (years) | | | | Total | Age Group (years) | | | | Total | |
SITE	18–24	25–44	45–64	65+	Men	18–24	25–44	45–64	65+	Women	Total
Panic (%)											
New Haven, Conn.	0.0	0.5	0.3	0.0	0.3	0.7	1.6	0.6	0.4	0.9	0.6
Baltimore	1.0	0.5	1.4	0.0	0.8	1.0	1.9	1.0	0.2	1.2	1.0
St. Louis	0.9	1.1	0.5	0.0	0.7	0.8	1.6	0.9	0.1	1.0	0.9
Obsessive-compulsive (%)											
New Haven	0.9	1.3	0.4	1.2	0.9	2.7	2.8	0.8	0.4	1.7	1.4
Baltimore	2.1	1.7	2.4	0.9	1.9	2.6	3.1	1.3	1.2	2.2	2.0
St. Louis	1.5	1.3	0.2	0.2	0.9	2.8	1.5	1.3	1.3	1.7	1.3

*DIS, Diagnostic Interview Schedule
Source: Myers JK, Weissman MM, Tischler GL et al: Six-month prevalence of psychiatric disorders in three communities. *Arch Gen Psychiatr* 41 (10): 962, 1984.

TABLE 2–21. Six-Month Prevalence of DIS/*DSM-III* Phobias by Sex and Age*

| | MEN | | | | | WOMEN | | | | | |
| | Age Group (years) | | | | Total | Age Group (years) | | | | Total | |
SITE	18–24	25–44	45–64	65+	Men	18–24	25–44	45–64	65+	Women	Total
Social phobia (%)†											
Baltimore	2.3	2.1	0.8	1.5	1.7	4.3	2.7	1.8	1.9	2.6	2.2
St. Louis	0.3	1.1	1.3	0.1	0.9	2.2	2.3	0.6	0.3	1.5	1.2
Simple phobia (%)											
New Haven, Conn.	3.1	3.1	4.5	0.7	3.2	6.3	8.5	4.2	3.6	6.0	4.7
Baltimore	9.3	5.8	8.4	6.1	7.3	18.1	16.0	15.6	12.5	15.7	11.8
St. Louis	2.1	2.2	2.8	1.5	2.3	5.6	10.2	4.5	1.9	6.5	4.5
Agoraphobia (%)											
New Haven	0.7	1.4	1.2	0.5	1.1	5.3	6.0	3.3	1.2	4.2	2.8
Baltimore	3.9	2.5	4.1	3.3	3.4	7.3	8.8	8.3	5.5	7.8	5.8
St. Louis	1.0	0.8	1.3	0.0	0.9	4.9	5.5	4.1	1.0	4.3	2.7
Total phobia (%)‡											
New Haven	3.1	3.3	4.8	1.2	3.4	9.1	11.3	5.3	4.6	8.0	5.9
Baltimore	10.7	6.9	10.0	7.6	8.6	18.9	18.6	17.3	14.2	17.5	13.4
St. Louis	2.5	3.0	3.3	1.5	2.8	8.4	11.2	5.3	2.6	7.7	5.4

*DIS, Diagnostic Interview Schedule
†Data on social phobia were not collected in DIS 2 employed in wave 1 in New Haven
‡Some persons had more than one phobic diagnosis, so individual diagnostic categories do not add up to the rates presented in "total phobia"
Source: Myers JK, Weissman MM, Tischler GL et al: Six-month prevalence of psychiatric disorders in three communities. *Arch Gen Psychiat* 41 (10): 1984.

TABLE 2–22. Six-Month Prevalence of DIS/*DSM-III* Somatization and Antisocial Personality Disorder by Sex and Age*

SITE	MEN					WOMEN					
	Age Group (years)				Total Men	Age Group (years)				Total Women	Total
	18–24	25–44	45–64	65+		18–24	25–44	45–64	65+		
Somatization disorder (%)											
New Haven, Conn.	0.0	0.0	0.0	0.0	0.0	0.2	0.3	0.2	0.0	0.2	0.1
Baltimore	0.0	0.0	0.0	0.0	0.0	0.0	0.5	0.0	0.0	0.2	0.1
St. Louis	0.0	0.0	0.0	0.0	0.0	0.6	0.3	0.2	0.0	0.3	0.1
Antisocial personality (%)											
New Haven, Conn.	1.2	1.0	0.3	1.1	0.8	0.6	0.6	0.0	0.0	0.3	0.6
Baltimore	0.9	3.4	0.2	0.0	1.5	0.1	0.3	0.0	0.0	0.1	0.7
St. Louis	4.6	2.9	0.3	0.0	2.1	1.6	0.6	0.0	0.0	0.5	1.3

*DIS, Diagnostic Interview Schedule
Source: Myers JK, Weissman MM, Tischler GL et al: Six-month prevalence of psychiatric disorders in three communities. *Arch Gen Psychiat* 41 (10): 1984.

TABLE 2–23. Percentage Distribution and Rate per 100,000 Civilian Population of Resident Patients in State and County Mental Hospitals at End of Year, by Diagnosis and Age: United States, 1969, 1974, and 1979

DIAGNOSIS AND AGE*	1969	1974	1979	1969	1974	1979	1969	1974	1979
	Number			Percentage distribution			Rate		
Personality disorders,									
total	7,737	5,813	3,356	2.1	2.7	2.4	3.9	2.7	1.5
Less than 18	1,057	571	508	0.3	0.3	0.4	1.5	0.8	0.8
18–44	4,607	4,149	2,326	1.2	1.9	1.7	6.7	5.3	2.6
45–64	1,609	845	365	0.4	0.4	0.3	3.9	1.9	0.8
65+	464	248	157	0.1	0.1	0.1	2.4	1.1	0.6

Diagnostic Groupings:	Diagnostic Codes
Mental retardation	310–315
Alcohol and drug disorders	291, 303, 309.13; 294.3, 304, 309.14
Organic brain syndromes (excluding alcoholism and drug)	290, 292, 293, 294 (except 294.3), 309.0, 309.2–309.9
Affective (formerly depression)	296, 298.0, 300.4
Schizophrenia	295
Other psychoses	297, 298.1–298.9, 299
Other neuroses	300.0–300.3, 300.5–300.9
Personality disorders	301
Other	
Preadult disorders	307.0–307.2, 308
Other mental disorders	302, 305, 306, 307.3–307.4
Social maladjustment	316–317
No mental disorder	318
Undiagnosed	Includes only patients who have been admitted for suspected mental disorders, but for whom a diagnosis has not yet been established.

*Age additions during year; age is reported as of the last birthday prior to addition.
Source: *Mental Health,* United States, 1983.

such tranquilizers as promazine and chlorpromazine.

Patients with schizoid personality exhibit behavior that is aloof, insecure, and fearful. The prodrome seems to be familial, and it occurs in 40% of schizophrenics before the onset of schizophrenia. With psychotherapeutic treatment, the prognosis is good. The passive-aggressive person avoids confrontation and expressing his feelings; he is sullen, aggressive, given to procrastination, and inefficient. He is often treated in group therapy.

The psychosociopath is impulsive; he requires gratification even when it runs counter to laws and customs. In the United States, the disorder is prevalent in men, especially those from low income groups. They resist rehabilitation, refusing to see anything wrong with their behavior. The behavior becomes less pronounced by age 50 years. An estimated 2% to 7% of psychosociopaths have had run-ins with the law. Explanations offered for the development of this narcissistic personality include child neglect, inconsistent parental response, substance abuse, and sexual promiscuity. The child's response to this type of parental behavior is an amoral attitude, lack of deep emotional ties with others, rebelliousness, temper tantrums, and cruelty to animals. Therapy involves tranquilizers, antidepressants, and encouragement to conform to acceptable social interaction.

MENTAL RETARDATION

The average IQ range is between 90 and 110 as measured by typical individual intelligence tests, such as the Stanford-Binet. Those with scores below 90 are considered to be retarded. Seventy-five percent of all mentally retarded with IQs above 50 are educable. Those with IQs between 21 and 50 are considered to be trainable, whereas those testing lower than 20 need lifelong custodial care.

The many causes of mental retardation include metabolic disorders, such as phenyketonuria (PKU); chromosomal abnormalities leading to forms of retardation, such as Down syndrome and cri-du-chat. Other retardation results from cranial pressure, maternal infections, prenatal malnutrition, birth trauma, postnatal injury, CNS infection, poisoning, and cerebral hemorrhage. Fifty percent of all cases are of unknown cause. The well-known Down syndrome accounts for only 1% of all retardation.

State-operated facilities, the number of retarded residents, their rate per 100,000 of general population, total annual admissions, and live releases from 1950 through 1982 are shown in Table 2–24.

The residence trend of the mentally retarded in public facilities between 1950 and 1982 is depicted in Figure 2–6.

TABLE 2–24. Mentally Retarded Residents of State-Operated Residential Facilities for the Mentally Retarded: 1950–1982

YEAR	FACILITIES	TOTAL RESIDENTS ON JUNE 30	RESIDENTS PER 100,000 IN GENERAL POPULATION*	TOTAL ANNUAL ADMISSIONS	LIVE RELEASES†
1950	96	129,399	86.1	12,233	5,531
1955	99	145,870	89.9	13,096	5,581
1960	108	163,730	91.9	14,701	6,451
1965	143	187,273	97.7	17,300	7,993
1966	154	191,987	99.3	14,998	9,268
1967	165	193,188	98.9	15,714	11,665
1968	170	192,520	97.7	14,688	11,675
1969	180	189,394	95.1	14,868	14,701
1970	190	186,743	92.6	14,985	14,702
1971	190	180,962	88.6	15,370	17,080
1972	210	181,035	87.2	NA	NA
1973	NA	173,775	82.9	NA	NA
1974	235	166,247	78.6	NA	NA
1975	NA	159,041	74.4	13,424	18,320
1976	244	157,134	73.8	NA	NA
1977‡	263	151,972	69.7	10,132	11,897
1978	257	143,721	65.2	10,508	15,088
1979	256	138,592	62.1	13,573	16,980
1980	252	131,721	58.4	4,745	11,973
1981‡	285	125,500	55.1	7,874	13,024
1982‡	279	118,982	51.8	9,798	12,523

NA; statistics not available.
*Base is the civilian resident population on July 1.
†Figures through 1975 represent live releases in excess of the number of readmissions; figures for 1975 and later are total live releases.
‡Figures include between 20 and 30 mental hospitals and mental health centers with some mentally retarded residents.
Source: 1950–1971, National Institute of Mental Health, and Social and Rehabilitation Service, as reprinted in U.S. Bureau of the Census, *Historical Statistics of the United States, Colonial Times to 1970*, Series B428-443; 1972–1974, R.C. Scheerenberger, under the sponsorship of the National Association of Superintendents of Public Residential Facilities for the Mentally Retarded, as reprinted in K. Charlie Lakin, *Demographic Studies of Residential Facilities for the Mentally Retarded: An Historical Review of Methodologies and Findings*, tables 5 and 6; 1975–1976, U.S. Office of Human Development Services, as reported in U.S. Department of Commerce, *Statistical Abstract of the United States, 1978*, table 177; 1977, R.C. Scheerenberger, as presented in Developmental Disabilities Project on Residential Services and Community Adjustment, Brief No. 3, *1977 National Summary Between Public and Community Residential Findings;* 1978–1980, Krantz, Bruininks and Clumpner, *Mentally Retared People in State-Operated Residential Facilities*, annual; 1981–1982, R.C. Scheerenberger, *Public Residential Services for the Mentally Retarded, 1982.*

Data on facilities and mentally retarded residents by state as of 1977 are shown in Table 2–25. North Dakota had the highest rate of mentally retarded residents at 203.6 per 100,000 population. Nevada, West Virginia, and Kentucky had the lowest rates.

The percentage of mentally retarded individuals living in public facilities, community facilities or foster homes by sex, age, and additional disability is shown in Table 2–26.

FIG. 2–6.   Mentally retarded residents of public residential facilities, 1950–1982

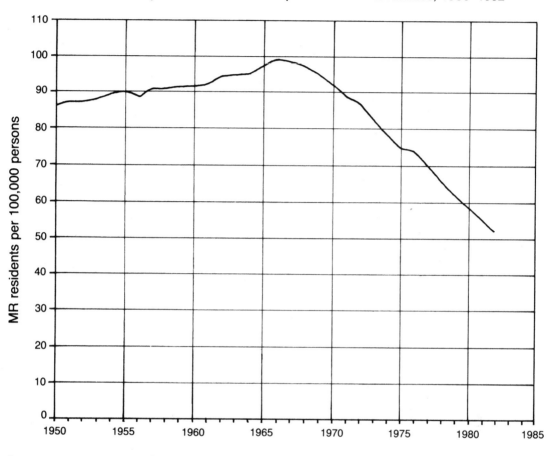

Source: *Digest of Data on Persons With Disabilities*, 1984. The National Institute of Handicapped Research, U.S. Dept. of Education.

The number of children in different care settings according to their degree of retardation and other limitations is presented in Table 2–27.

The number of mentally retarded children covered by the Education for All Handicapped Children Act by state is compared with other types of handicapped children in Table 2–28.

TABLE 2-25. Facilities and Mentally Retarded Residents in Public Residential Facilities and Community Residential Facilities, by State: 1977

STATE	FACILITIES		MENTALLY RETARDED RESIDENTS			Mentally retarded residents per 100,000 civilian residential population
	Public residential facilities	Community residential facilities	Public residential facilities	Community residential facilities	Total	
United States, total	263	4,427	151,972	62,397	214,369	99.1
New England						
Maine	3	46	496	629	1,125	103.7
New Hampshire	1	18	664	105	769	90.6
Vermont	1	64	438	220	658	136.3
Massachusetts	9	157	5,581	1,848	7,429	128.5
Rhode Island	1	15	756	181	937	100.3
Connecticut	12	52	3,279	947	4,226	136.0
Middle Atlantic						
New York	21	167	18,134	3,314	21,448	119.7
New Jersey	8	84	7,946	789	8,735	119.2
Pennsylvania	17	354	9,473	6,102	15,575	132.2
East North Central						
Ohio	11	124	6,542	2,485	9,027	84.3
Indiana	6	42	3,289	479	3,768	70.7
Illinois	14	147	6,320	6,076	12,396	110.2
Michigan	12	474	6,318	4,126	10,444	114.4
Wisconsin	3	116	2,359	2,084	4,443	95.5
West North Central						
Minnesota	8	176	3,017	3,140	6,157	154.9
Iowa	2	45	1,432	1,150	2,582	89.6
Missouri	5	193	2,166	2,663	4,829	100.6
North Dakota	2	12	1,145	185	1,330	203.6
South Dakota	2	21	835	260	1,095	158.9
Nebraska	3	87	1,155	937	2,092	134.0
Kansas	4	102	1,443	1,089	2,532	108.8
South Atlantic						
Delaware	1	6	546	89	635	109.1
Maryland	6	26	2,926	374	3,300	79.7
District of Columbia	1	2	923	40	963	139.6
Virginia	5	51	4,076	508	4,584	89.3
West Virginia	4	9	822	56	878	47.2
North Carolina	6	74	3,659	643	4,302	77.8
South Carolina	4	27	3,617	310	3,927	136.6
Georgia	8	31	2,807	306	3,113	61.7

TABLE 2-25. Continued

STATE	FACILITIES		MENTALLY RETARDED RESIDENTS			Mentally retarded residents per 100,000 civilian residential population
	Public residential facilities	Community residential facilities	Public residential facilities	Community residential facilities	Total	
Florida	6	172	4,503	2,342	6,845	81.0
East South Central						
Kentucky	2	18	607	950	1,557	45.1
Tennessee	3	84	2,079	903	2,982	69.4
Alabama	4	17	1,791	207	1,998	54.1
Mississippi	4	13	1,666	354	2,020	84.5
West South Central						
Arkansas	5	16	1,682	215	1,897	88.5
Louisiana	8	20	3,617	1,256	4,873	124.3
Oklahoma	3	7	1,978	584	2,562	91.2
Texas	3	88	11,919	2,280	14,199	110.7
United States, total	263	4,427	151,972	62,397	214,369	99.1
Mountain						
Montana	2	61	321	438	759	99.8
Idaho	1	21	453	266	719	83.9
Wyoming	1	12	533	101	634	156.2
Colorado	3	72	1,539	848	2,387	91.2
New Mexico	2	34	547	206	753	63.3
Arizona	3	26	973	343	1,316	57.3
Utah	1	14	849	412	1,261	99.5
Nevada	3	5	166	30	196	30.9
Pacific						
Washington	6	115	2,450	1,550	4,000	109.4
Oregon	2	65	1,781	811	2,592	109.1
California	9	772	9,725	6,870	16,595	75.5
Alaska	1	14	105	119	224	55.0
Hawaii	1	59	524	177	701	78.4

Source: Developmental Disabilities Project on Residential Services and Community Adjustment, Brief No. 3. *1977 National Summary Between Public and Community Residential Findings*, table 2 and figure 6.

TABLE 2–26. Mentally Retarded Persons in Residential Programs, by Sex, Age, Other Diagnostic Condition and Type of Facility: 1977

CHARACTERISTICS (PERCENT OF TOTAL)	PUBLIC RESIDENTIAL FACILITIES	COMMUNITY RESIDENTIAL FACILITIES	FOSTER HOMES
Total residents	151,972	62,397	4,999
Sex			
Male	57.2	55.3	46.3
Female	42.8	44.7	53.7
Age			
0–4	0.7	2.4	3.4
5–9	0.5	6.4	5.8
10–14	1.3	10.0	3.6
15–21	25.4	19.3	18.5
22–39	46.2	38.5	25.9
40–62	21.5	19.9	31.2
63+	4.3	3.5	11.8
Other condition			
Deaf	3.6	2.7	3.7
Blind	6.1	3.2	2.6
Epilepsy	32.5	17.5	8.0
Cerebral palsy	19.3	8.7	4.0
Autistic traits	4.2	2.9	2.6

Source: *Digest of Data on Persons With Disabilities,* 1984. The U.S. National Institute of Handicapped Research.

TABLE 2–27. Mentally Retarded Persons in Residential Programs, by Degree of Retardation and Functional Limitation: 1977

CHARACTERISTICS (% OF TOTAL)	PUBLIC RESIDENTIAL FACILITIES	COMMUNITY RESIDENTIAL FACILITIES	FOSTER HOMES
Total residents	151,972	62,397	4,999
Degree of retardation:			
Borderline	1.7	8.1	8.1
Mild	7.4	22.9	21.0
Moderate	15.6	35.9	37.5
Severe	27.8	22.2	27.1
Profound	47.3	10.8	6.1
Limitations*			
Cannot walk	25.6	10.7	4.1
Is not toilet trained	13.6	12.2	4.9
Cannot dress self	55.8	21.1	11.1
Cannot feed self	11.4	11.2	4.6
Does not understand language	6.9	7.4	4.2
Cannot talk	16.3	19.6	13.5

*Percentages do not add to 100. A resident may have multiple limitations or none.
Source: *Digest of Data on Persons With Disabilities,* 1984. The National Institute of Handicapped Research, U.S.

ORGANIC BRAIN SYNDROME

Generally, organic brain syndrome is described as irreversible diffuse brain damage. It often has a slow insidious onset and deteriorates to dementia and delirium. The most common form of irreversible damage is caused by Alzheimer's disease. Fifty percent of all organic brain damage is of this form. Another 30% is senile dementia related to cerebrovascular impairment. The remaining 20% of all cases can be caused by such conditions as syphilis, poisoning, and head injury. About 20% of the population over age 80 years suffers from some form of organic brain syndrome.

Of the estimated 4 million people with organic brain damage, 1.5-2 million have Alzheimer's disease. It is caused by the degeneration of the nerve cells in the outer layer of the brain. Cells are sparser in the affected brain than in the normal brain, and remaining cells are frequently abnormal. At present, the disease is incurable. The cause is unknown. Research efforts, however, are focused on the production of acetylcholine in the brain. This enzyme is diminished in patients with Alzheimer's disease, especially in the hippocampus and frontal lobe. Blood flow and glucose utilization are also greatly reduced in the patient with Alzheimer's disease. The disease may also be related to one's genetic encoding, or it may be caused by a slow-acting virus. Aluminum is also being explored as a cause of this disease.

Vascular dementia, or multiple infarct dementia, accounts for the next most common dementia. Atherosclerotic disease causes plaques to build up in brain vessels, or they may become blocked by emboli that prevent blood circulation to the brain. Cells in the deprived area die, and the classic symptoms of dementia develop.

Signs of organically caused mental deterioration include impaired abstract thinking, disorientation, limitation on memory and imagination, loss of humor, a disregard for personal hygiene, and apathy. Patients may be depressed, uninhibited, irritable, and anxious. In severe instances, they may hallucinate, exhibit incoherent speech, and be restless or stuporous.

Diagnosis involves evaluating the patient's medical history, EEG or CT scans, neurologic tests that measure intellectual functioning, and tests of liver, thyroid, and renal function. Treatment is usually supportive except when impairment is due to an ascertainable physical cause, such as renal insufficiency, underactive thyroid, brain tumor, poisoning, or vitamin B12 deficiency—to name just a few. When the NIMH surveyed St. Louis, Baltimore, and New Haven for the lifetime prevalence in the noninstitutionalized population of the severely cognitively impaired, the prevalence was at or just above 1% (Table 2–29).

TABLE 2–28. Children Ages 3–21 Served Under the Education for all Handicapped Children Act and Aid to States for Handicapped Children, by Handicapping Condition and State: 1981–1982 School Year

STATE	SPECIFIC LEARNING DISABLED	SPEECH IMPAIRED	MENTALLY RETARDED	SERIOUSLY EMOTIONALLY DISTURBED	ORTHO-PEDICALLY IMPAIRED	DEAF AND HARD OF HEARING	VISUALLY HANDI-CAPPED	DEAF AND BLIND	MULTI-HANDI-CAPPED	OTHER HEALTH IMPAIRED	TOTAL
United States, total*	1,624,989	1,136,309	786,775	339,629	57,967	74,694	29,174	2,486	71,289	79,519	4,202,831
New England:											
Maine	8,349	6,055	5,019	4,317	446	473	142	17	788	341	25,947
New Hampshire	8,001	2,221	1,660	1,209	166	368	217	7	141	189	14,179
Vermont	4,382	2,418	2,917	451	259	321	119	12	516	168	11,563
Massachusetts	49,382	32,175	29,656	19,165	1,538	1,889	768	143	3,074	1,957	139,747
Rhode Island	11,212	3,498	1,610	1,209	205	242	69	12	171	207	18,435
Connecticut	29,489	13,996	7,081	12,328	478	1,219	693	5	0	1,022	66,311
Middle Atlantic:											
New York	69,489	40,883	40,541	47,933	5,747	4,631	1,839	113	6,171	33,057	250,404
New Jersey	59,251	63,752	14,794	15,529	1,422	2,324	1,355	46	3,736	1,477	163,686
Pennsylvania	57,727	63,327	46,828	14,816	1,939	4,286	1,934	8	26	28	190,919
East North Central:											
Ohio	71,657	62,112	61,279	6,135	3,346	2,660	964	145	2,147	0	210,445
Indiana	25,126	40,727	25,092	2,539	808	1,324	520	30	1,186	295	97,647
Illinois	87,718	77,335	43,707	31,780	4,584	4,160	1,803	108	1,512	3,088	255,795
Michigan	52,311	45,361	28,150	19,293	4,575	3,104	909	0	349	9	154,061
Wisconsin	26,861	17,714	13,874	9,095	1,122	1,320	466	53	648	440	71,593
West North Central:											
Minnesota	35,249	19,231	14,289	5,013	1,299	1,468	422	41	0	904	77,916
Iowa	22,347	15,218	12,238	4,127	800	1,009	229	40	701	185	56,894
Missouri	36,155	32,722	21,066	7,136	942	1,214	401	65	531	699	100,931
North Dakota	4,137	3,281	1,939	326	165	209	78	21	08	56	10,212
South Dakota	3,048	5,312	1,490	339	243	454	98	41	435	62	11,522
Nebraska	12,422	9,626	6,191	1,761	520	734	211	0	347	0	31,812
Kansas	15,809	13,576	6,966	3,614	304	758	265	28	746	478	42,544
South Atlantic:											
Delaware	6,520	2,191	2,140	2,807	288	253	142	39	4	56	14,440
Maryland	49,171	25,053	9,069	3,444	923	1,595	604	54	2,935	448	93,296
District of Columbia	1,916	1,252	1,289	685	99	490	54	24	203	117	6,129
Virginia	36,139	31,010	17,676	6,398	840	1,905	1,878	55	3,278	392	99,571
West Virginia	12,851	11,946	11,177	1,235	393	513	277	21	247	894	39,554
North Carolina	45,448	25,644	36,788	5,010	1,054	2,299	681	32	1,991	1,094	120,041
South Carolina	18,855	18,829	23,500	5,285	757	1,131	492	12	415	200	69,476
Georgia	35,274	28,806	29,110	16,523	653	2,034	838	61	1,011	1,469	115,779
Florida	55,782	43,530	25,963	14,931	1,973	2,065	787	94	2,371	2,342	149,838

TABLE 2–28. Continued

STATE	SPECIFIC LEARNING DISABLED	SPEECH IMPAIRED	MENTALLY RETARDED	SERIOUSLY EMOTIONALLY DISTURBED	ORTHO-PEDICALLY IMPAIRED	DEAF AND HARD OF HEARING	VISUALLY HANDI-CAPPED	DEAF AND BLIND	MULTI-HANDI-CAPPED	OTHER HEALTH IMPAIRED	TOTAL
East South Central:											
Kentucky	18,127	24,528	22,717	2,193	657	1,125	524	133	1,200	853	72,057
Tennessee	39,410	32,823	20,629	2,623	1,101	2,406	778	9	1,554	1,126	102,459
Alabama	19,868	14,924	34,402	3,880	357	1,057	413	55	1,053	388	76,397
Mississippi	14,435	16,207	16,828	397	395	646	258	43	247	0	49,456
West South Central:											
Arkansas	18,539	10,976	17,244	633	417	696	310	20	770	259	49,863
Louisiana	34,354	20,970	16,927	4,643	536	1,681	422	75	938	1,333	81,879
Oklahoma	28,312	20,117	13,009	960	372	836	299	42	1,179	353	65,479
Texas	141,924	66,286	29,326	15,432	3,200	4,870	1,821	215	14,242	4,557	281,873
Mountain:											
Montana	6,497	4,475	1,449	569	88	253	177	28	640	103	14,279
Idaho	8,222	4,067	2,795	543	338	404	164	17	222	382	17,154
Wyoming	4,980	3,082	998	785	184	160	44	49	423	139	10,844
Colorado	20,937	8,303	6,041	7,358	835	1,030	333	68	1,242	0	46,147
New Mexico	12,319	5,307	2,805	1,948	337	412	149	36	1,054	87	24,454
Arizona	25,376	11,527	6,270	5,148	903	1,036	400	0	777	700	52,137
Utah	13,246	7,571	3,164	10,245	316	741	337	37	1,745	182	37,584
Nevada	6,672	2,924	1,211	541	214	193	82	1	352	266	12,456
United States, total*	1,624,989	1,136,309	786,775	339,629	57,967	74,694	29,174	2,486	71,289	79,519	4,202,831
Pacific:											
Washington	30,137	13,312	9,892	4,573	1,072	1,274	354	48	1,837	1,417	63,916
Oregon	22,236	11,835	4,905	2,546	981	1,455	576	31	131	582	45,278
California	190,727	92,594	29,874	9,163	7,296	7,213	2,341	203	5,445	15,032	359,888
Alaska	6,135	3,010	780	316	198	244	51	22	190	61	11,007
Hawaii	7,897	1,728	1,674	437	257	405	73	26	181	0	12,678
Bureau of Indian Affairs†	2,561	942	736	263	25	106	13	1	187	25	4,859

*Totals exclude children residing outside the 50 states and the District of Columbia and thus differ slightly from the totals reported in table III.A.1.
†The Bureau of Indian Affairs in the U.S. Department of the Interior administers the special education programs in Bureau-operated schools; these programs are not under the authority of individual States, and the children served by these programs are not included in the state statistics.
Source: Office of Special Education and Rehabilitative Services, U.S. Department of Education; statistics reported by state agencies under P.L. 94-142 and P.L. 89-313; published in *Annual Report to Congress on the Implementation of Public Law 94-142*, 1983.

Those suffering from organic brain syndrome—excluding brain damage caused by alcohol and drugs—constitute about 10% of the institutionalized population in state and county mental facilities (Table 2–30). The greatest proportion of this 10% is age 65 years or older.

TABLE 2–29. Six-Month Prevalence of Cognitive Impairment by Sex and Age

	MEN					WOMEN					
	Age Group (years)				Total	Age Group (years)				Total	
SITE	18–24	25–44	45–64	65+	Men	18–24	25–44	45–64	65+	Women	Total
Severe (%)											
New Haven, Conn.	0.7	0.6	0.8	6.3	1.4	0.3	0.1	1.4	4.2	1.2	1.3
Baltimore	0.0	0.0	1.1	5.7	1.1	0.4	0.5	1.1	4.8	1.4	1.3
St. Louis	0.4	0.2	0.8	4.6	1.0	0.9	0.3	0.7	3.6	1.1	1.0
Mild (%)											
New Haven	1.7	0.7	6.3	11.5	4.0	2.1	1.4	3.8	11.6	4.1	4.0
Baltimore	2.7	2.1	9.7	14.2	6.2	0.9	1.7	4.5	16.6	5.2	5.7
St. Louis	4.0	2.5	5.2	18.4	5.5	1.6	2.5	9.2	15.0	6.2	5.9

Source: Myers JK, Weissman MM, Tischler GL et al: Six-month prevalence of psychiatric disorders in three communities. *Arch Gen Psychiatr* 41 (10): 1984.

TABLE 2–30. Percentage Distribution and Rate per 100,000 Civilian Population* of Resident Patients Diagnosed with Organic Brain Syndrome in State and County Mental Hospitals at End of Year, by Diagnosis and Age: United States, 1969, 1974, and 1979

DIAGNOSIS† AND AGE‡	1969	1974	1979	1969	1974	1979	1969	1974	1979
	Number			Percentage distribution			Rate		
Organic brain syndrome, total	77,752	34,706	23,127	21.0	16.1	16.6	39.0	16.4	10.4
Less than 18	1,149	570	284	0.3	0.3	0.2	1.6	0.8	0.4
18–44	9,009	4,506	2,934	2.4	2.1	2.1	13.2	5.8	3.3
45–64	20,096	8,663	5,142	5.4	5.0	3.7	48.6	19.9	11.6
65+	47,498	20,967	14,767	12.8	9.7	10.6	241.4	95.0	58.8

Sources: *National Institute of Mental Health.* Unpublished data from the Survey and Reports Branch, Division of Biometry and Epidemiology (1969, 1974, 1979).
Notes: The data in this table, which are provided by the State agencies of mental health through the *Annual Census of Patient Characteristics, State and County Mental Hospital Inpatient Services, Additions and Resident Patients,* are reported for the fiscal year used by the particular State. For most States, it is the year ending June 30. These data will differ slightly from numbers of inpatient additions shown in table 2.7 that are based on responses to the *Inventory of Mental Health Facilities* by individual State and county mental hospitals, which are given the option to report on either a calendar- or fiscal-year basis. Information on the "State" hospital in Puerto Rico is excluded.
*The populations used in the calculations of these rates are estimates of the U.S. civilian populations (provided by the Bureau of the Census and published in Series P-25 publications) as of July 1 for each respective year.
†*Diagnostic Classification* The diagnostic classification can be found in *Diagnostic and Statistical Manual of Mental Disorders* (Second Edition), American Psychiatric Association, 1968. The codes corresponding to the diagnostic categories shown in the tables are as follows:
Diagnostic Groupings   Diagnostic Code
Organic brain syndromes (excluding alcoholism and drug)   290, 292, 293, 294 (except 294.3), 309.0, 309.2–309.9
‡Age additions during year (age is reported as of the last birthday at end of reported year).

Alcohol Abuse 3

A lcohol abuse is often a response to stress and is classified as a mental disease by the International Classification of Diseases. Persons with low self-esteem are especially susceptible.

ALCOHOL

The most commonly abused substance in the United States is alcohol. In the United States, 7% of all adults age 18 years and older—roughly 10 million people—are problem drinkers. Alcohol consumption is estimated by sales figures and survey reports, which question individuals sampled about their drinking habits.

By 1981, the average volume of ethyl alcohol imbibed was 2.77 gallons, or 6.9 gallons of 80 proof liquor per person. These figures are higher than pre-Prohibition levels. Consumption since Prohibition has been rising steadily although the rate of increase in the early 1980s was slower than that of previous years (Figure 3–1).

Per capita sales have increased by 35% since the 1960s but by only 7% since 1971. Since 1971 beer sales rose 22%, wine rose 13%, and distilled-spirits sales fell 10%.

Although the alcoholic thinks of his or her abuse as a personal weakness that affects no one else, the facts are otherwise. In 1977,

FIG. 3–1.   Trends in apparent consumption of ethyl alcohol in gallons per person

Ethyl alcohol total

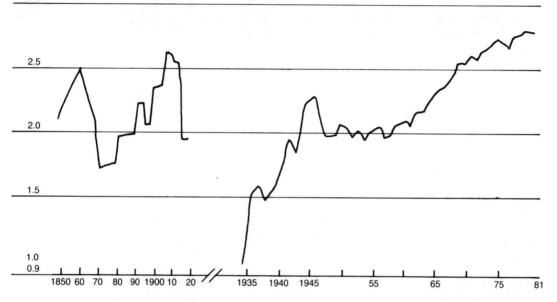

Source: *Public Health Reports*, Vol. 98, No. 5, Sept. 1983.

alcohol abuse cost the United States an estimated $49.4 billion directly and indirectly. These costs were for medical treatment, motor vehicle damage, fire damage, and lost productivity. The costs in lives lost and the pain and suffering experienced by those who live with the consequences of alcohol abuse are incalculable.

In 1980, investigators interested in the benefits of company-sponsored alcohol treatment studied the pioneer program of the New York Telephone Company. The company was saving as much as $1.5 million annually. Before the program, untreated alcoholic employees missed on average 60 "work days" annually and accounted for $2,000 in medical costs for injuries and physical debility because of their alcohol abuse.

About 10% of all deaths in the United States are from alcohol abuse; many of the fatalities result from fires and motor-vehicle accidents. [One-half of all highway deaths are related to alcohol consumption.] In 1981, the death rate due to motor vehicle accidents involving drivers with blood alcohol levels of 0.10% or higher was 4.7. Other deaths as previously pointed out, are homicides, particularly among family members and close associates. Depression is common among alcoholics, so alcohol is involved in suicides as well.

Chronic alcoholism is a chief cause of cirrhosis. Indeed cirrhosis still ranks as the ninth leading cause of death, accounting, as of 1982, for 63,000 deaths annually. Alcohol consumption is also associated with cancer of the liver, pancreas, esophagus, and mouth.

MEN VS WOMEN

Until recently, alcohol abuse was regarded as essentially a man's disease; most rehabilitation and medical efforts were directed toward male clients. The social stigma in the United States associated with the female alcoholic contributed to concealment of the problem. Thus, numbers projected for female alcoholics are underestimates. Today, however, it is known that between 1.5 and 2.25 million women have serious drinking problems; 27% of all women who drink are problem drinkers. Annual alcohol-related deaths among females are estimated at 50,000. This includes deaths from cirrhosis, accidents, suicide, and the other causes already mentioned.

Particular concern centers on alcohol consumption among pregnant women, for excessive alcohol consumption during pregnancy can lead to fetal alcohol syndrome. This can trigger, among other complications, retardation and even death, for the infant. Because alcohol crosses the placental barrier, the fetus may well have blood levels of alcohol similar to those of its mother.

Recent surveys indicate that 73% of all women are aware of the dangers of drinking while pregnant and reduce their alcohol consumption when pregnant. About 61% of pregnant women reported abstaining from alcohol; the 12% of nonpregnant women who were moderate-to-heavy drinkers declined to 2% when they became pregnant. Nevertheless, the number of babies born with fetal alcohol syndrome remains at 1 to 3 per 1,000 live births.

As Table 3–1 shows, men abuse alcohol much more than do women (although the percentage of women who drink heavily is not miniscule as once thought). On the positive side, men seem to have reduced their consumption since the mid-1970s. The data show large percentages of men and women who are either abstemious or temperate. Results from the 1970s' surveys show these data to be rather constant—roughly one-third of the population is abstemious, another one-third consists of light drinkers who consume less than 0.21 ounces of absolute alcohol (less than half a drink) daily on average. The remaining one-third are moderate drinkers (0.22 to 0.99 ounces, or up to 1 drink a day) or heavy drinkers (1 ounce or more, i.e., two drinks daily).

The finding that fewer people are drinking is not inconsistent with increased alcohol consumption, however, because the smaller percentage of people still drinking are drinking more wine and beer than previously.

THE AGE OF DRINKERS

The pattern of alcohol use is one also of greater consumption by the young. Between 1974 and 1982, alcohol use by adults age 18 to 25 years was about 22% greater than among adults 26 years and older. But adults age 26 years and older reported higher daily consumption. In 1982, about 12% of this older age group said it drank 20 or more days each month. Of those age 18 to 25 years, 68% reported

TABLE 3–1. Alcohol Consumption Status of Persons Age 18 Years and Older, According to Sex: United States, selected years 1971–79 (data are based on interviews of samples of the noninstitutionalized population)

SEX AND ALCOHOL CONSUMPTION	YEAR						
	1971	1972	1973	1974	1975	1976	1979
Total				Persons (%)			
Abstain	36	36	34	36	36	33	33
Light	34	32	29	28	31	38	34
Moderate	20	23	23	28	21	19	24
Heavy	10	10	14	11	12	10	9
Male							
Abstain	30	28	25	24	27	26	25
Light	29	29	24	24	27	33	29
Moderate	26	28	29	34	26	24	31
Heavy	15	15	22	13	20	18	14
Female							
Abstain	42	44	42	42	45	39	40
Light	40	34	35	32	35	44	38
Moderate	13	18	17	21	15	15	18
Heavy	5	4	6	5	4	3	4

Note: Alcohol consumption status is defined in ounces of absolute alcohol (ethanol) consumed per day as follows: abstain, 0; light, .01–.21; moderate, .22–.99; and heavy, 1.00 or more.
Source: Clark WB, Midanik L, Knupfer G: *Report on the 1979 National Survey*. University of California. Contract No. ADM 281-77-0021. Prepared for the National Institute of Alcohol Abuse and Alcoholism. Rockville, Md., December 1981.
Source: *Health, 1983*

having imbibed alcohol during the month before the 1982 survey, while 57% of older adults reported recent consumption as did 27% of youths. The percentages in each age group reporting that they had ever used alcohol were high: 94.6% for young adults, 88.2% for older adults, and 65.2% for youths ages 12 to 17 years.

CONSUMPTION PATTERNS

The number of days in the month just before the survey during which respondents of different ages consumed alcohol is shown in Table 3–2.

Since the late 1970s, drinkers younger than 22 years are inbibing less. The age group older than 22 years does not show a decline.

Future trends in alcohol consumption can be judged in part by reviewing the frequency of alcohol consumption among teenagers. In recent years, investigators have been paying much more attention to patterns among this youngest portion of the population.

When surveyed, the percentage of high school seniors who reported drinking heavily was higher for males than females. The rate for both has remained fairly constant from the mid-1970s through 1982. Since the mid-1970s, about 6% of all high school seniors report daily alcohol use, 70% report use within the last month, and 93% report having tried alcohol at some time before being surveyed.

During the 1978–1982 surveys, about 10% of children questioned reported that they had drunk alcohol by the sixth grade. Thirty percent of the 1981 graduating class had drunk alcohol by the

TABLE 3–2. Patterns of Alcohol Use (youth, young adults, and older adults, 1982)

	1	2	3
DAILY CONSUMPTION	YOUTH: (12–17 years) (1581) (%)	YOUNG ADULTS: (18–25 years) (1283) (%)	OLDER ADULTS: (26+ years) (2760) (%)
Days Used in Past Month:			
20 or more	*	6.5	11.4
5–19	5.9	28.2	18.2
3–4	6.7	11.4	9.7
1–2	13.8	21.8	17.1
Not past month user	38.3	26.7	31.5
Not sure	*	*	*
Never used	34.8	5.4	11.8

Note: Some categories do not add to 100% because of rounding.
*Less than 0.5%.
Source: Alcohol, Drug Abuse and Mental Health Administration

FIG. 3–2.   Trends in lifetime prevalence for earlier grade levels based on retrospective reports from seniors, 1969–81

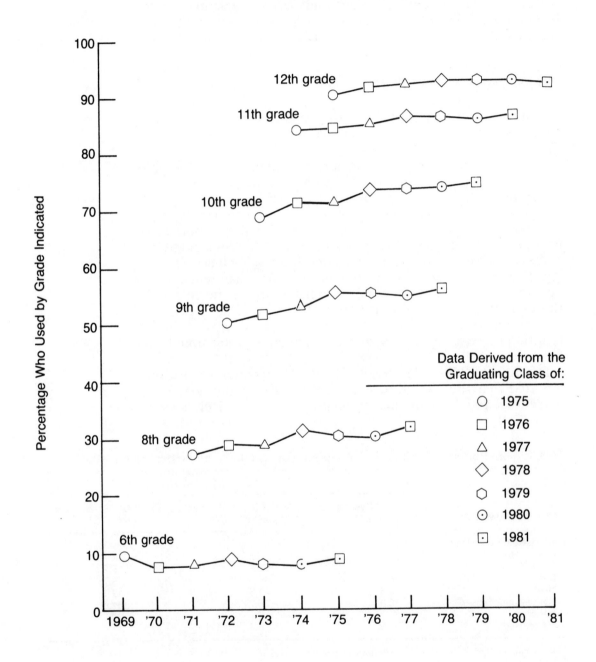

Source: Alcohol, Drug Abuse and Mental Health Administration.

eighth grade, 56% during the ninth grade, and 75% during the tenth grade. As mentioned, 93% reported some consumption of alcohol by the time they were high school seniors. The trend in consumption of alcohol by respondents age 12 through 17 years from 1969 through 1981 is graphed in Figure 3–2.

The problem of teenage alcohol use and abuse should ease as national programs to educate school officials and parents about the dangers of alcohol abuse begin to show the results of heightened awareness. The first such major program began in October 1982. It was followed by another in 1983 that emphasized treatment programs for youth. Other groups, both government and privately sponsored, have organized to educate youth about the dangers of drinking and driving.

Between 1977 and 1978, the percentage of teenage drivers ages 16 to 19 years who drove with measurable levels of alcohol in their blood rose from 20% to 28%. This same 8% increase occurred also in older drivers. Since behavior often follows what people think, periodic surveys are taken to determine attitudes toward drug use. They show that disapproval of drinking is rising (Figure 3–3).

ALCOHOLISM

Any individual whose drinking leads to the loss of a job, friends, or a marriage and who cannot stop drinking is an alcoholic. Further, the alcoholic has developed a physical and psychologic dependency. Physical dependency is particularly apparent in the withdrawal syndrome that alcoholics develop when they try to stop drinking. Symptoms include tremors, neurological seizures and various other unpleasant physical reactions to alcohol deprivation.

Current scientific belief holds that some people have an inherited disposition to become alcoholic. One researcher investigating the genetic link reviewed 39 studies of the genetic question conducted over the past 4 decades. He noted that alcoholics matched with nonalcoholic cohorts, were more likely to have an alcoholic parent, sibling, or distant relative.[1] But the nature/nurture effects are particularly difficult to sort out since alcohol use may also be culturally determined or patterned in the family. Thus, the environment seems to play some role in the development of alcoholism.

The same review found that in several studies at least 45% of alcoholic subjects did not have an alcoholic relative.

In the 1970s, researchers such as Goodwin in Denmark compared

---

[1]Cotton NS: The familial incidence of alcoholism. *Studies on Alcohol* 40: pp. 89–116, 1979.

the adopted sons of alcoholics with those of nonalcoholics. He found that the former were three times as likely to become alcoholics as the latter.[2] The children of alcoholics were also likely to become alcoholic at an early age to a degree that required treatment.

During a second phase of the Goodwin study, children of alcoholics who were adopted by nonalcoholic adults were compared with siblings brought up by their alcoholic parents. The nonadopted siblings raised by alcoholic parents were no more likely to become alcoholic than their siblings who were raised in a nonalcoholic environment. The investigators concluded that exposure to an alcoholic environment did not increase the likelihood of genetically susceptible individuals to become alcoholic. One can also look at this study in the reverse direction; the findings suggest that being brought up in a nonalcoholic environment did not lead to less alcoholism in genetically disposed individuals.

In 1980, researchers at the University of Iowa found a correlation between childhood behavioral problems and alcoholism in later life among adoptees. But there was no correlation to psychiatric problems in their biologic parents or to other environmental factors in their adoptive homes. In light of this and other studies, childhood behavioral problems, including hyperactivity, seem to be predictors of alcoholism in later life just like alcoholic relatives.

Current opinion tends to the view that a genetic factor influences the development of alcoholism in 35% to 40% of all alcoholics. This factor is linked with physiologic characteristics that individually vary. Some of these characteristics still being investigated include the sensitivity of the brain to alcohol, the blood alcohol elimination rate, and the propensity both to develop a tolerance to alcohol and to develop physical dependence on alcohol.

EFFECTS

A noticeable sign of alcoholism is the tolerance and dependence that develops in the chronic drinker; the effects of alcohol felt by a light drinker after one or two cocktails will not be felt by the alcoholic until he or she has imbibed much more alcohol—perhaps as much as one pint of whiskey. At the same time, the symptoms of withdrawal from alcohol, which can include tremors and neurologic seizures, appear in the chronic drinker if he does not keep the

---

[2]Goodwin DW et al: Alcohol problems in adoptees raised apart from biological parents. *Arch Gen Psychiat* 28: pp 238–243, 1973.

FIG. 3–3.   Trends in disapproval of licit drug use for seniors, parents, and peers, 1975–1981

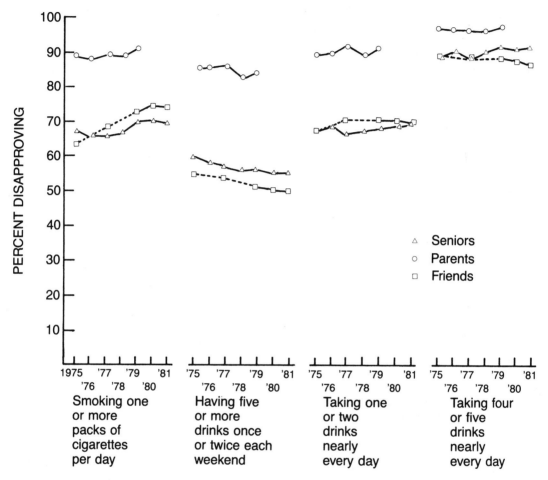

Note: Points connected by dotted lines have been adjusted because of lack of comparability of question-context among administrations.

Source: Alcohol, Drug Abuse and Mental Health Administration.

concentration of alcohol in his blood at high levels. The alcoholic also shows signs of impaired cognitive functioning. Young alcoholics commonly perform like elderly people on tests of cognitive skills, memory, reflex reaction, and motor coordination.

Alcoholic dementia is characterized by destruction of cerebral cortical neurons in the frontal lobe. Yet, some studies revealed that after detoxification, alcoholics had restored ability, especially if they were young; this finding, however, has not always been replicated.[3,4] Chronic organic brain syndromes caused by alcoholism are the second most common of the known causes of adult dementia; they cause 10% of such syndrome symptoms, whereas Alzheimer's disease accounts for 50%.

Other toxic effects of chronic alcohol consumption include liver damage; this may deteriorate to cirrhosis leading to death when the liver can no longer function. Before this occurs, other organs can become impaired when the liver inadequately metabolizes and detoxifies metabolites in circulating blood. Alcohol in the blood can itself have a deleterious effect on the cardiovascular, nervous, and endocrine systems.

Noticeable endocrine effects are seen in the feminization of men when chronic alcohol consumption lowers their production of androgens. They suffer decreased libido and infertility and assume a more feminine appearance. Women similarly can experience ovarian dysfunction.

Another serious effect of alcohol consumption is its association with several cancers, including cancer of the stomach, large intestine, pancreas, and liver. But long before the development of cancer, alcoholics frequently suffer from nutritional deficiencies and anemia. Drinking fills them with empty calories, and they often do not feel hunger that would ordinarily prompt them to eat food that is nutritious.

Excessive drinking can lead to psychiatric illnesses, sometimes as a direct result of alcohol's psychopharmalogic activity. Numerous studies find a higher incidence of depression, anxiety, hysteria, sociopathic behavior, drug abuse, and anorexia nervosa in alcoholics then in nonalcoholics. But it is not always clear whether alcohol causes all these conditions or whether they lead to alcohol consumption. A causative influence can flow in either direction.

The latter has important implications for treatment. Hypothesizing that alcohol consumption has caused these other problems requires that a person's alcohol problem be solved before other alcohol-related problems can be addressed. On the other hand, alcoholism probably cannot be arrested until underlying psychological problems that have led to alcoholism are ameliorated.

---

[3]Ron MA, Acker W, Shaw GK et al: Computerized tomography of the brain in chronic alcoholism—a survey and follow-up study. *Brain* 105: pp 497–514, 1982.
[4]Adams KM, Granl I, Reed R et al: Neuropsychology in alcoholic men in their late thirties. One-year follow-up. *Am J Psychiat* 137: pp 928–931, 1979.

DIAGNOSIS

The intellectual and psychological changes that occur in chronic drinkers offer one avenue of detection and diagnosis. Various screening tests are now in use in several countries. They can determine whether one has a drinking problem. One of the best known tests used in the United States is the Michigan Alcoholism Screening Test (MAST). It consists of 25 true or false statements that address the typical medical, social, and behavioral problems of excessive drinking. When evaluated, this test proved successful in distinguishing between a known group of alcoholic men and a nonalcoholic group.[5] Such tests are, however, vulnerable to false responses that alcoholics in denial may offer. Results depend on the respondents' veracity. Laboratory tests can be used in conjunction with the questionnaire when a physician suspects that a patient has a drinking problem.

Researchers have also identified some biochemical markers in the blood of alcoholics that can identify a chronic drinker. One is serum gamma-glutamyl transpeptidase (GGTP). Although the result of testing for GGTP may be affected by other drug use and liver abnormality, marker tests together with other routine blood chemistry tests can accurately differentiate the alcoholic from the nonalcoholic. As physical ailments become clinically manifested, cirrhosis of the liver, e.g., diagnosis becomes easier.

TREATMENT

Several forms of therapy are used. Depending on the patient's mental and physical impairment, treatment includes hospitalization for detoxification so that withdrawal trauma and physical conditions created by alcohol consumption can be medically treated. Other treatment consists of counseling to promote effective coping with stress.

Certain physiologic responses occur in the alcoholic when he is confronted with the sight and smell of alcohol. Hence, treatment may consist of aversion therapy in which imbibing alcohol is accompanied by unpleasant stimuli.

In other therapy, the alcoholic is exposed to the sight and smell of alcohol without imbibing until alcohol-related stimuli are not as strongly associated with its consumption. Because relapse occurs so often in detoxified alcoholics, some investigators suggest that aversion or neutralizing conditioning be an essential part of all

---

[5]Brady JP, Foulks ET, Childress AR et al: The Michigan Alcoholism Screening Test as a survey instrument. *J Operational Psychiat*, 31(1): pp 27–31, 1982.

alcoholic rehabilitation.[6]

An aversion drug often used to stabilize a recovering alcoholic is Antabuse. It blocks the enzyme, aldehyde dehydrogenase, which mediates the metabolism of alcohol by the liver into acetaldehyde and then into carbon dioxide and water. Patients receiving Antabuse who imbibe alcohol accumulate high serum levels of acetaldehyde. The chemical can cause nausea, flushing, hypertension, and heart failure if the alcohol and Antabuse levels are sufficiently high. Although Antabuse helps to promote abstinence, its use can be dangerous, and those treated often fail to take their medication and relapse. Patients beginning Antabuse therapy must be free of any alcohol for 12 hours before the first dose is administered. They must also be aware of the alcohol that may be present in medications and ordinary aftershave that can be absorbed through the skin.

Another substance being explored for the same purpose is lithium because of its beneficial effects in treating other affective disorders. Compliance is still a problem, however, as it is with any medication.

One of the best known treatments for alcoholism is membership in the organization Alcoholics Anonymous (AA). The strength of this form of treatment is the peer support given to the alcoholic and the nonjudgmental approach to the alcoholic's problem. Other offshoots of AA, such as Alateen, can help the alcoholic's family as well.

Many forms of treatment for the alcoholic can be given in either an inpatient or outpatient setting. In recent years there has been a growing inclination to treat in an outpatient setting because the cost is lower. But definitive research on the effectiveness of treating alcoholics as outpatients has not determined the question. Similarly, some studies, particularly the Rand study, indicate that alcoholics can drink moderately after detoxification without relapsing. Follow-up studies reveal that the subjects who did not relapse may not have been as dependent on alcohol as most chronic alcoholics. Four years after therapy, alcoholics who drank moderately had relapsed into more severe alcoholism than those who had been abstemious after detoxification. Similarly, whether one is treated as an outpatient or inpatient depends mainly on the severity of one's dependency on alcohol and one's overall physical and mental health.

In 1976, the Association of Halfway House Alcoholism Programs conducted a survey of programs available to alcoholics. Nine

---

[6]Hinson R E, Siegel S: *Alcohol Tolerance and Dependence.* Amsterdam: Elsevier/North Holland Biomedical, pp 181–199, 1980.

TABLE 3–3. Distribution of Clients in Treatment by Facility Location in Units Providing Alcoholism Treatment Only and Units Providing Combined Alcoholism and Drug Abuse Treatment (National Drug and Alcoholism Treatment Utilization Survey, September 30, 1982)

FACILITY	ALCOHOLISM ONLY		COMBINED		TOTAL	
	Number	(%)	Number	(%)	Number	(%)
Hospital	32925	16.2	5980	6.9	38905	13.5
Quarterway House	1599	0.8	367	0.4	1966	0.7
Halfway House/Recovery Home	14398	7.1	1805	2.1	16203	5.6
Other Residential Facility	14938	7.4	4257	4.9	19195	6.6
Outpatient Facility	136322	67.2	71941	83.4	208263	72.0
Correctional Facility	2735	1.4	1944	2.3	4679	1.6
Total	202917	100.0	86294	100.0	289211	100.0

Source: Alcohol, Drug Abuse and Mental Health Administration

TABLE 3–4. Demographic Characteristics of Clients in Units Providing Alcoholism Treatment Only and Units Providing Combined Alcoholism and Drug Abuse Treatment (National Drug and Alcoholism Treatment Utilization Survey, September 30, 1982)

CLIENT CHARACTERISTICS	ALCOHOLISM ONLY		COMBINED		TOTAL	
	Number	(%)	Number	(%)	Number	(%)
Race/Ethnicity:						
American Indian	7622	3.8	2916	3.4	10578	3.7
Asian	649	.3	273	.3	922	.3
Black	32010	16.0	12255	14.6	44265	15.6
Hispanic	22155	11.1	4419	5.2	26574	9.3
White	137016	68.6	63814	76.2	200830	70.9
Total	199492	100.0	83677	100.0	283169*	100.0
Sex:						
Male	156333	78.7	60991	75.0	217324	77.6
Female	42294	21.2	20262	24.9	62556	22.3
Total	198627	100.0	81253	100.0	279880*	100.0
Age (years):						
18 and under	8042	4.0	5641	6.9	13683	4.9
19–20	11698	5.9	6465	8.0	18163	6.5
21–44	116198	59.0	47609	59.0	163807	59.0
45–59	46630	23.6	15923	19.7	62553	22.5
60–64	9872	5.0	3310	4.1	13182	4.7
65+	4381	2.2	1733	2.1	6114	2.2
Total	196821	100.0	80681	100.0	277502*	100.0

*Data on race/ethnicity were reported for 97.7% of the total 289,933 reported clients; data on sex were reported for 96.5% of all clients and on age for 95.7% of them.
Source: Alcohol, Drug Abuse and Mental Health Administration

percent, or 161 programs, were designed only for women; 56% were for men only, and 35% were coeducational with 10% to 30% of beds reserved for women. A treatment utilization survey taken in 1982 indicated that 202,917 people underwent treatment for alcoholism, 86,294 for alcoholism combined with drug abuse (Table 3–3). Most of them went to outpatient facilities in 1982.

The second greatest provider of treatment is the inpatient hospital. Alcoholism treatment was also provided to 63,000 clients in residential facilities, one-half of them being halfway houses or recovery homes. Most clients of alcoholism treatment centers were white males. The characteristics of clients of alcohol-treatment and drug-treatment programs are summarized in Table 3–4. The location of treatment facilities and programs is summarized in Table 3–5. Programs are distributed throughout urban, suburban, and rural areas.

Funding for alcohol treatment programs comes from many sources both private and governmental (Figure 3–4).

TABLE 3–5. Principal Population Served in Units Providing Alcoholism Services Only and Units Providing Combined Alcoholism and Drug Abuse Services (National Drug and Alcoholism Treatment Utilization Survey, September 30, 1982)

	ALCOHOLISM ONLY		COMBINED		TOTAL	
POPULATION*	Number	(%)	Number	(%)	Number	(%)
Inner City	587	21.5	167	11.0	754	17.8
Other Urban	990	36.3	511	34.0	1501	35.5
Suburban	535	19.6	249	16.6	784	18.5
Rural	617	22.6	577	38.4	1194	28.2
Total	2729	100.0	1504	100.0	4233	100.0

*The area where the majority of the clients served by a unit reside.
Source: Alcohol, Drug Abuse and Mental Health Administration

FIG. 3–4. Alcoholism treatment funding by source

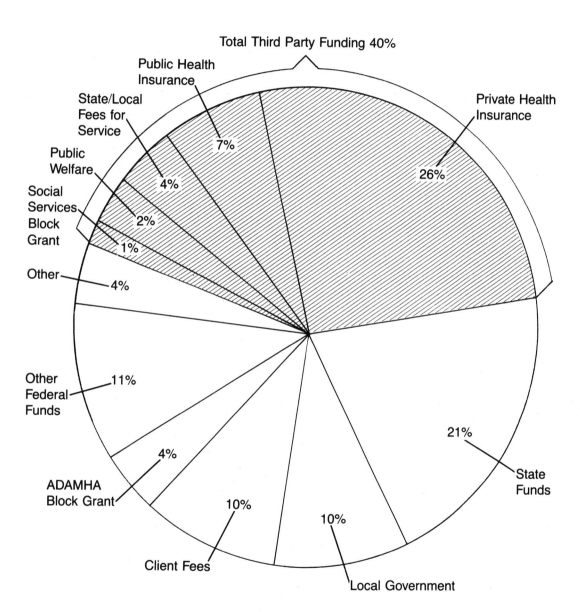

Total Reported Funding: $1,123,175,000
(3997 Units)

Source: NDATUS, Sept. 30, 1982.

4 Other Drug Use and Abuse

Alcohol is often used in conjunction with other drugs, especially by the young who smoke marijuana and drink. Drugs commonly abused or illegally used alone or in combination with alcohol include narcotics, hallucinogens, prescription drugs, over-the-counter remedies, barbiturates, and amphetamines.

Currently, 20 million people are estimated to use marijuana; 4 to 5 million use cocaine, and 22 million report that they have tried cocaine at least once. Drug related deaths reported quarterly for 1978 in each region are shown in Table 4–1. Much attention has been given to the sudden upsurge in drug abuse that developed from the mid-1960s to the 1980s in the United States and other Western countries; drug use history, nevertheless, varies considerably. Some drugs have been used for centuries for religious or medicinal purposes, or both. Many others have only been synthesized or discovered since 1935.

MARIJUANA

Marijuana is *cannabis sativa*, the name given internationally to drug derivatives of the Indian hemp plant. The active hallucinogenic agent in cannabis is a resin produced by the plant called tetrahydrocannabinol, more commonly called THC. The plant is

TABLE 4–1. Average Number of Drug-Related Deaths per Quarter by Drug and Region, 1978 (regional drug situation analysis)

SUBSTANCE	NATIONWIDE	NORTHEAST		NORTH CENTRAL		SOUTHEASTERN		SOUTH CENTRAL		WESTERN	
		Boston SMSA	New York SMSA	Chicago SMSA	Detroit SMSA	Atlanta SMSA	Wash. D.C. SMSA	Dallas SMSA	Denver SMSA	Los Angeles SMSA	San Francisco SMSA
Heroin	142	2	15	20	14	1.5	2	2.0	0.5	41	16
Cocaine	11	*	–	0.8	0	0.25	0.25	–	0.8	–	0.8
Hallucinogens	20	2	0.3	2.3	0.8	0	0	–	–	7.8	1.8
Stimulants	67	4	6	4.5	1.3	1	3	2.8	2.0	14	8
Depressants	406	12	50	–	–	5.5	–	–	–	–	–

*Indicates no listing for that drug type, or no deaths for that drug type.
Source: Alcohol, Drug Abuse and Mental Health Administration

prepared in several ways in different parts of the world to form substances known, inter alia, as marijuana, hashish, charas, ghanja, dagga, kef, and bhang. Hashish and charas are made from the pure resin and are considerably stronger than the derivative known in the United States. The substance used in India called bhang is the least potent of the various preparations.

Cannabis was used in Asia and central China by 3000 B.C. and almost as early in India and the Near East. It may have been introduced into Europe by way of North Africa. In the 20th century, marijuana use in the United States spread from the lower classes to intellectuals and then filtered down to university students in the 1960s and 1970s. This was followed by fad use among high school and grade school students. Although cannabis was regarded as a medicinal drug historically, its modern use centers on its mind-altering effects. Marijuana is more familiarly known as "pot," "grass," and "tea."

Although THC is fat-soluble and remains in animal tissue for months after marijuana use ceases, it is not physically addicting because heavy users do not experience physical withdrawal symptoms as do alcoholics and opiate addicts. But users can experience psychological dependence. This is most readily discernible in the pattern of its use, which is repetitive and regular.

Smoking marijuana can induce dizziness, lightheadedness, heaviness in the limbs, reduced coordination and movement, irritation of the eyes and mouth, quickened heart beat, and tinitis or the hearing of other sounds. Toxic absorption leads to motor restlessness, hallucinations, and delusions. Psychologically, users may feel euphoric, experience disruption of their thought processes and memory, and develop disturbance in their ability to judge distances and to accurately organize spatial relationships. Loss of contact with reality is not uncommon and is attended by anxiety, fear, or panic.

National drug use surveys taken during the 1970s showed marked increases in use. The percentage of American young adults, age 18 to 25 years, reporting that they had used marijuana (referred to as the "prevalence of use") increased from 48% in 1972 to 68% in 1979. But the 1982 survey showed a slight decline; only 64.1% reported at least one use of marijuana.

Similarly, by 1982 use declined among youngsters age 12 to 17 years to 26.7%, down from 30.9% in 1979. During the 1970s, prevalence had risen continuously. Prevalence among older adults ages 26+ years continues to increase in the 1980s. But it must be remembered that the cohort moving into this age range is the same one that was the youth group in the 1970s, which showed sharp increases in use. Members of this group are simply bringing their history with them as they move into the older adult statistical category.

The recency pattern, indicated by use within 1 month of surveys from 1979 to 1982, shows a dramatic drop in use among youths and young adults. In the late 1970s, nearly 16.7% of all persons 12 to 17 years reported recent marijuana use. This figure fell to 11.5% by 1982. Trend analysis for recent marijuana use among persons age 12 to 17 years according to sex, race, population density, and geographic region is shown in Table 4–2. Recency of use since 1971 is greater for males than females, for whites than nonwhites, for youngsters in large metropolitan centers, and, until the late seventies, for youngsters in the west and northeastern states. In 1982, the geographic trend changed when use in the north central states equalled that in the northeast and was greater than that in the west where the decline became marked.

The pattern of recent marijuana use among young adults ages 18 to 25 years from 1976 to 1982 is shown in Table 4–3. Again, more males were recent users than females and more whites than nonwhites until 1982. Then, the rate for whites fell significantly; the rate for blacks did not fall. Interestingly, through 1979 those with the least education, the non-high school graduate, and those who attended 1 to 3 years of college reported the most recent marijuana use. By 1982, persons with more education showed a

TABLE 4–2. Past Month Use of Marijuana (in %) Among Subgroups of Youth: 1971–1982

SUBGROUP	1971	1972	1974	1976	1977	1979	1982	Change: 1979–'82*
Youth: (age 12–17 years):	6	7	12	12.3	16.6	16.7	11.5	SSS
Sex:								
Male	7	9	12	14	20	19	13	SS
Female	5	6	11	11	13	14	10	S
Race:								
White	†	8	12	12	17	17	12	SS
Black and other races	†	2	9	11	14	15	10	NS
Region:								
Northeast	9	7	14	13	22	20	15	NS
North Central	5	7	11	16	20	19	15	NS
South	2	4	6	7	8	12	8	$
West	11	14	19	17	22	16	10	$
Population density:								
Large metropolitan	9	†	14	18	22	20	17	NS
Small metropolitan	7	†	11	11	17	14	8	S
Nonmetropolitan	3	†	10	8	10	15	9	SS

*Significance levels: SSS, 0.001; SS, 0.01; S, 0.05; $, 0.10; NS, not significant.
†Not tabulated.
Source: National Drug Abuse Institute

TABLE 4–3. Past Month Use of Marijuana (in %) Among Subgroups of Young Adults: 1976–1982

SUBGROUP	1976	1977	1979	1982	Change: 1979–'82*
Young adults (age 18–25 years):	25.0	27.4	35.4	27.4	SSS
Sex:					
Male	31	35	45	36	SS
Female	19	20	26	19	SS
Race:					
White	26	28	36	26	SSS
Black and other races	22	24	34	35	NS
Education:					
Non-high school graduate	23	21	41	35	NS
High school graduate	21	29	30	26	NS
Attended college:	32	30	38	24	SSS
Completed 1–3 years	33	32	40	26	SSS
Graduate	28	22	33	19	S
Now a full-time college student	32	31	37	26	S
Region:					
Northeast	26	34	40	31	$
North Central	27	29	38	27	SS
South	18	17	30	26	NS
West	35	33	36	27	$
Population density:					
Large metropolitan	29	31	39	32	$
Small metropolitan	28	29	36	26	SS
Nonmetropolitan	16	18	30	23	S

*Significance levels: SSS, 0.001; SS, 0.01; S, 0.05; $, 0.10; NS, not significant.
Source: Alcohol, Drug Abuse and Mental Health Administration

lowered use as did the least educated. But their relative positions had changed: the least educated were the highest percentage of recent users.

By the late 1970s, recent use was highest in the northeast followed by the north central states. As with young users, the group reporting recent use was highest in large metropolitan areas and lowest in nonmetropolitan ones.

Among older adults ages 26+ years, recent use was greatest among blacks, much more among males than females, more among college graduates and those who attended college, and moderately greater in the west and northeast than in other regions. As before, recent use was greater in large metropolitan areas. (Table 4–4).

The pattern of marijuana use in 1982 by age is shown in Table 4–5. Its use in combination with alcohol and details about its frequency of use are also summarized. Users age 18 to 25 years who were teenagers and preteenagers in the 1970s have used marijuana more than those older and those who are currently younger. They

TABLE 4–4. Past Month Use of Marijuana (in %) Among Subgroups of Older Adults: 1976–1982

SUBGROUP	1976	1977	1979	1982	Change: 1979–'82*
Older adults (age 26+ years):	3.5	3.3	6.0	6.6	NS
Sex:					
Male	6	4	9	10	NS
Female	2	2	3	3	NS
Race:					
White	3	3	6	6	NS
Black and other races	6	4	8	9	NS
Education:					
Non-high school graduate	1	1	3	2	NS
High school graduate	3	3	5	5	NS
Attended college:	6	7	10	11	NS
Completed 1–3 years	5	9	9	11	NS
Graduate	7	4	11	11	NS
Region:					
Northeast	5	5	7	9	NS
North Central	2	3	4	5	NS
South	3	1	5	5	NS
West	4	5	9	9	NS
Population density:					
Large metropolitan	5	5	8	9	NS
Small metropolitan	4	3	6	6	NS
Nonmetropolitan	1	1	4	3	NS

*Significance levels: SSS, 0.001; SS, 0.01; S, 0.05; $, 0.10; NS, not significant.
Source: Alcohol, Drug Abuse and Mental Health Administration

also used it more with alcohol than the others and more frequently. Many persons age 18 to 25 years reported in 1982, however, that they had not used marijuana in the past month. Those working to educate the public about the hazards of mind alteration through substance use and abuse have directed much of their efforts to reaching the young and to trying to determine the reasons and conditions surrounding the introduction of drugs to the young. Surveys of high school seniors asked them to report when they first tried marijuana (Figure 4–1).

The graduating class of 1981 reported trying marijuana in the sixth grade in a slightly higher percentage than preceding graduating classes. The symbols representing each class at the sixth grade level show a slight increase from 1969 though 1975. Those in the eighth grade in 1973 and 1974, who became the high school seniors of 1977 and 1978, show the most abrupt increase in marijuana use.

Figure 4–1 shows that each class during the 1970s had more members trying and or using marijuana at each grade level. When the seniors of 1981 were in the sixth grade, e.g., about 3% had tried marijuana; by the eighth grade 15% had tried it; by the tenth grade

TABLE 4–5. Marijuana Use (in %): Youth, Young Adults, and Older Adults, 1982

PATTERNS	YOUTH (age 12–17)*	YOUNG ADULTS (age 18–25)*	OLDER ADULTS (age 26+)*
Lifetime Frequency of Use:			
1 or 2 times	7.7	9.5	6.2
3 to 10 times	7.2	12.6	5.0
11 to 99 times	5.7	17.4	4.9
100 or more times	5.4	24.0	6.9
Not sure how many times	0.7	0.6	*
Never used marijuana	73.3	35.9	77.0
Alcohol Use on Same Occasion:			
Usually	3.9	15.6	5.3
About one-half the time	3.3	8.1	3.5
Occasionally/rarely	9.4	27.3	7.1
Never	9.6	10.0	5.9
Not sure if same occasion/skipped	†	3.0	1.3
Never used marijuana	73.3	35.9	77.0
"Daily" Marijuana Use:			
Ever used on 20+ days in one month	5.8	21.2	4.2
All other users	20.9	42.9	18.8
Never used marijuana	73.3	35.9	77.0
Current Patterns (days used in past month):			
20 or more	2.1	7.0	1.1
5–19	3.5	8.7	2.1
3–4	1.3	3.1	1.2
1–2	4.2	8.0	2.2
Not past month user	15.1	36.6	16.4
Not sure how many days	†	0.6	†
Never used marijuana	73.3	35.9	77.0

*Some categories do not add to 100% because of rounding.
†Less than 0.5%.
Source: Alcohol, Drug Abuse and Mental Health Administration

FIG. 4–1.   Marijuana: trends in lifetime prevalence for earlier grade levels based on retrospective reports from seniors, 1969–1981

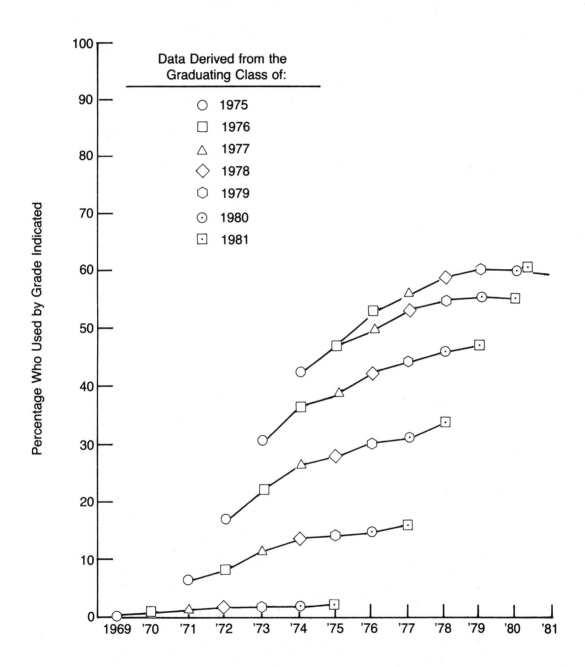

Source: Alcohol, Drug Abuse and Mental Health Administration.

45% had tried it; and by the twelfth grade about 60% had tried it.
This was slightly less than the percentage of the previous classes of
1979 and 1980. These data clearly show the early points of
marijuana introduction into the lives of many American young
people. They also show that marijuana use behavior has been
fluctuating.

The trend in perceived harmfulness among young people during
the 1970s and early 1980s is shown in Figure 4–2. As of 1978,
youngsters in increasing numbers believed that smoking marijuana, especially the daily use of marijuana, was harmful. Interesting-

FIG. 4–2.   Trends in perceived harmfulness: marijuana and cigarettes, 1975–1981

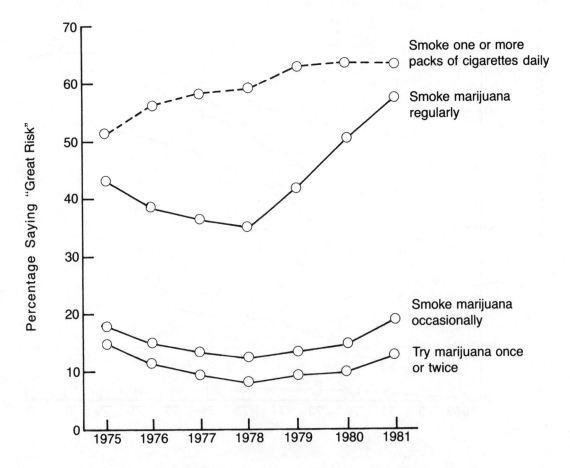

Source: Alcohol, Drug Abuse and Mental Health Administration.

FIG. 4–3. Trends in disapproval of illicit drug use for seniors, parents, and peers, 1975–1981

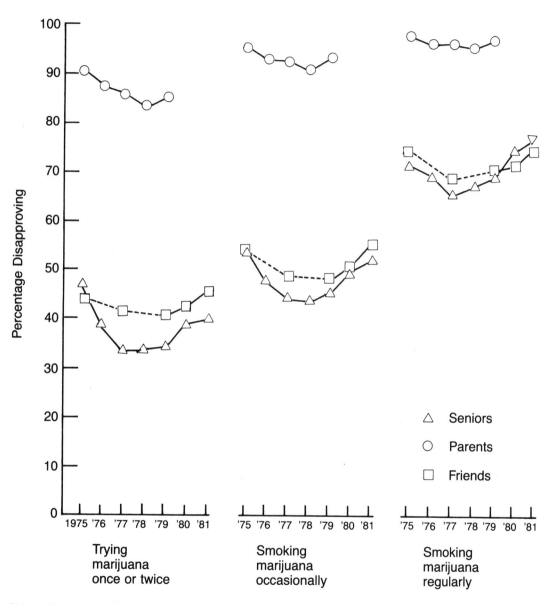

Note: Points connected by dotted lines have been adjusted because of lack of comparability of question-context among administrations. (See text for discussion.)

Source: Alcohol, Drug Abuse and Mental Health Administration.

ly, throughout the period, large numbers of them also felt that smoking cigarettes was harmful. This belief also shows a wider acceptance by 1979. Over the past decade, the trend in parental and peer disapproval of marijuana perhaps shows more clearly than anything else the reason for the recent decline in its use. Disapproval has increased among each group markedly although the relative differences between groups remain as parents continue to disapprove more than their children (Figure 4–3). The gap between them has closed with respect to frequent use of marijuana as they each disapprove more than not.

The actual number of marijuana users are identified by sex, race, and residence for 1977 and projected to 1995 (Table 4–6).

OPIATES

Before passage of the Harrison Act in 1914, morphine and heroin were legal. Opium was first modified into morphine in the 1800s. It was used so widely as a pain reliever in the Civil War that morphine addiction became known as the "soldier's disease." Diacetylmorphine, developed in 1890, is more commonly known as heroin. It was hailed as an improved form of morphine, one that could relieve pain without adverse effects. It was added to cough medicines and other medicinal elixirs including much touted alcoholism remedies. Alcoholics did indeed find relief from their drinking problem by being in a perpetual state of heroin stupor! By 1900, nearly 1 million persons were heroin addicts.

Addictions to heroin and other narcotics develop easily as both mind and body adapt. Withdrawal of these substances causes physiologic reactions including muscle pain, vomiting, diarrhea, and convulsions that may lead to death. As with alcohol, physiologic adaption to narcotics also causes increased tolerance. Hence, addicts need either to increase dosage or to take the drug in a more direct way to achieve the desired euphoria. They may change routes of administration from inhalation to IV injection "mainlining."

By the mid-1980s, heroin overdosing claimed 10,000 lives. Many addicts receive methadone, a synthetic narcotic that reportedly reduces the desire for heroin and blocks the euphoria it generates. To date, methadone clinics are more successful in helping older addicts, who desire to turn their lives around, than they have been in helping younger heroin addicts.

Another successful method is encouraging addicts to live in drug-free residence centers where peer pressure and professional counseling enable them to steer clear of drugs. Some of the better known ones established in the 1970s are Synanon and Phoenix House.

Heroin use in 1982 was concentrated in people age 18 to 25 years. In 1979, 3.5% reported that they had tried heroin. Less than one-half as many in the 18- to 25-year age range reported trying heroin in 1982; less than 0.5% of those younger than 18 years in 1979 reported trying heroin (Table 4–7). The trend in use of heroin and other opiates by sex for 1975 through 1981 is shown in Figure 4–4.

The percentage of young people who first use heroin or another opiate or both at various grade levels beginning with the senior class of 1975 when they were in the sixth grade is presented in Figures 4–5 and 4–6. For the most part, introduction to heroin does not appear to take place until the ninth and tenth grades, but. students start to use other opiates in the eighth grade (Figure 4–5).

Projections on young adults who will be using heroin through 1995 based on trends in the late 1970s are presented in Table 4–8.

TABLE 4–6. Young Adults 18 to 25 Using Marijuana Currently, 1977 Survey, and Projections for 1985, 1990, and 1995*

SUBGROUPS OF YOUNG ADULTS*	1977	1985	1990	1995
Females	3,382	3,308	2,995	2,766
Males	5,786	5,652	5,124	4,747
Whites	7,925	7,603	6,771	6,160
Nonwhites	1,166	1,262	1,243	1,234
Large Metropolitan Residents	4,056	3,964	3,591	3,321
Other Metropolitan Residents	2,908	2,842	2,575	2,381
Nonmetropolitan Residents	1,848	1,807	1,638	1,514

*Numbers are in thousands and based on 1977 prevalence rates.
Source: Alcohol, Drug Abuse and Mental Health Administration

TABLE 4–7. Lifetime Prevalence of Heroin, 1972–1982: Youth, Young Adults, and Older Adults

FREQUENCY	1972	1974	1976	1977	1979	1982	Change: 1979–'82†
Youth (age 12–17 years):	(880)	(952)	(986)	(1272)	(2165)	(1581)	
Ever used	0.6%	1.0%	0.5%	1.1%	0.5%	‡	—
Young adults (age 18–25 years):	(772)	(849)	(882)	(1500)	(2044)	(1283)	
Ever used	4.6%	4.5%	3.9%	3.6%	3.5%	1.2%	SS
Older adults (age 26+ years):	(1613)	(2221)	(1708)	(1822)	(3015)	(2760)	
Ever used	‡	0.5%	0.5%	0.8%	1.0%	1.1%	NS

Note: Numbers in parenthesis indicate size of sample.
*From 1972 through 1982, prevalence of past month heroin use has been less than 0.5% in each major age group.
‡Less than 0.5%.
†Significance levels: SSS, 0.001; SS, 0.01; S, 0.05; $, 0.10; NS, not significant.
Source: Alcohol, Drug Abuse and Mental Health Administration

FIG. 4–4. Trends in annual prevalence of 15 drugs by sex, 1975–1981

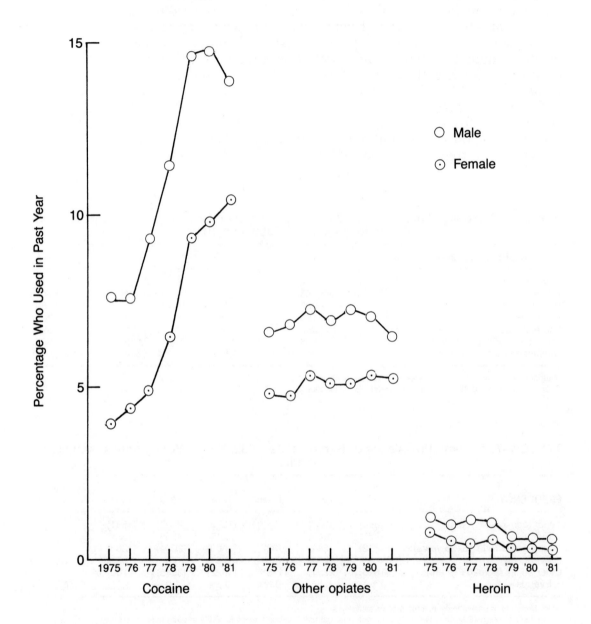

Source: Alcohol, Drug Abuse and Mental Health Administration.

FIG. 4–5.   Heroin: trends in lifetime prevalence for earlier grade levels based on retrospective reports from seniors, 1969–1981

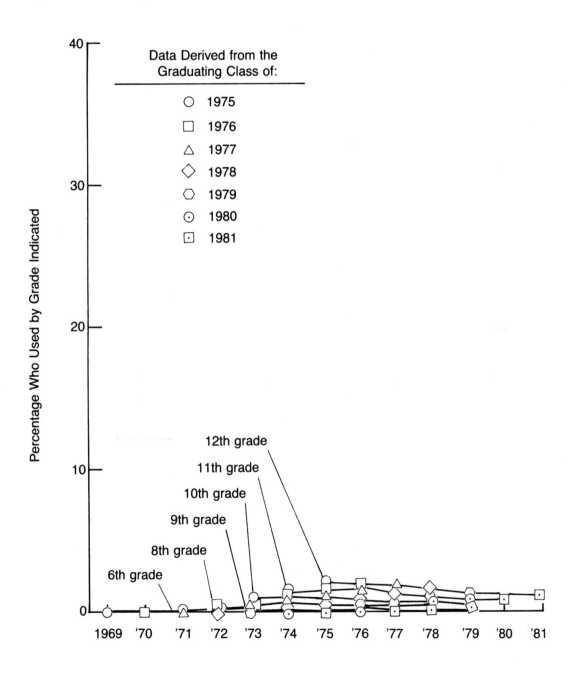

Source: Alcohol, Drug Abuse and Mental Health Administration.

FIG. 4-6. Other opiates: trends in lifetime prevalence for earlier grade levels based on retrospective reports from seniors, 1969–1981

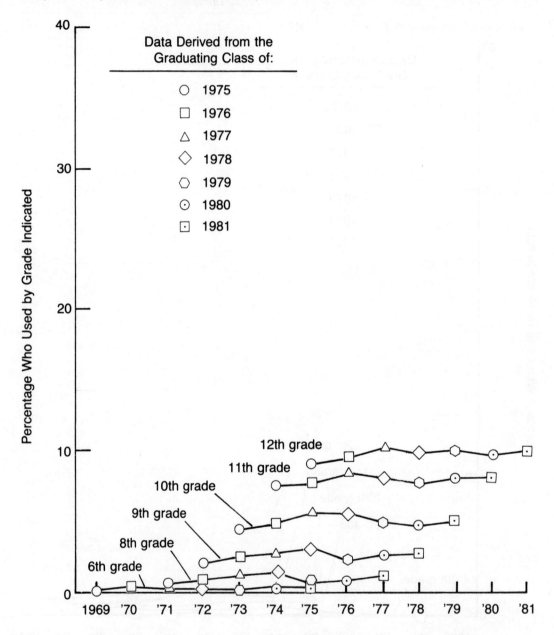

Source: Alcohol, Drug Abuse and Mental Health Administration.

TABLE 4–8. Young Adults 18 to 25 in Various Subgroups Using Heroin Currently, 1977 Survey, and Projections for 1985, 1990, and 1995

SUBGROUPS OF YOUNG ADULTS	1977	1985	1990	1995
Females	—	—	—	—
Males	115*	113	102	95
Whites	84	80	72	65
Nonwhites	39	42	41	41
Large Metropolitan Residents	38	37	34	31
Other Metropolitan Residents	49	48	44	40
Nonmetropolitan Residents	—	—	—	—

*Numbers are in thousands and based on 1977 prevalence rates.
Source: Alcohol, Drug Abuse and Mental Health Administration

TABLE 4–9. Lifetime Prevalence of PCP, 1976–1982: Youth, Young Adults, and Older Adults

AGE GROUP	EVER USED (in %)				
	1976	1977	1979	1982	Change: 1979–'82*
Youth (age 12–17 years):	3.0	5.8	3.9	2.2	S
Young adults (age 18–25 years):	9.5	13.9	14.5	10.5	SS
Older adults (age 26+ years):	0.7	1.1	2.2	2.4	NS

*Signficance levels: SSS, 0.001; SS, 0.01; S, 0.05; $, 0.10; NS, not significant
Source: National Institute on Drug Abuse

HALLUCINOGENS

Marijuana has been classified as a hallucinogen. But often it is treated separately from other hallucinogens because of its widespread use. Other hallucinogens are LSD-25—a form of ergot, mescaline derived from the peyote plant in the southwestern United States and Mexico, psilocin derived from Mexican mushrooms, and phencyclidine (PCP).

The physiologic effects of these drugs vary; each varies from person to person and in the same person on different occasions. The effects of psilocin are evident within 30 minutes and last 5 to 6 hours; LSD's effects become apparent within 60 minutes and last from 8 to 10 hours to several days.

The drugs mentioned usually cause vivid, unusual and usually unreal sensory experiences. Users experience detachment and depersonalization from their own body and their surroundings. Some users who experience "bad trips" are frightened by the sensations the drug induces and have a psychotic-like reaction that can last months and require hospitalization. These drugs can trigger mood swings, and time and space distortion; they can be particularly dangerous if users attempt to drive while under their influence.

Physiologically, these drugs act like central nervous system (CNS) stimulants. They elevate systolic blood pressure, and excite the CNS and brain. Hallucinogens are not thought to be physiologically addictive because users do not develop withdrawal symptoms. But they are considered to be psychologically addictive and can cause total preoccupation when used repeatedly. Tolerance develops quickly and seems to be cross-transferable. This feature suggests that all the hallucinogens operate similarly in the brain.

Natives of the western hemisphere have been using mescaline for 2,000 years, often for religious rites. But the use of hallucinogens, especially LSD, in the United States began in the 1950s. By 1960, intellectuals, artists, creative types, psychologists, and even medical investigators were using these drugs. Initial research seemed to indicate that they could cause chromosomal damage, but results are still incomplete. The rise in suicide rate among users, heightened awareness of the psychotic and adverse effects, and knowledge that in high doses these drugs are lethal have led to a fall in their use. Mortality statistics connected with PCP abuse are particularly sobering. Trends since 1975 in the use of hallucinogens, generally, LSD, and PCP are graphically shown in Figure 4–7.

The 1982 Drug Abuse and Mental Health Administration drug use survey showed a fall in hallucinogen use since 1979. The youngest age group and the group of users older than age 35 years have tried these drugs much less than young adults between 18 and 35 years. Falls in the use of hallucinogens are apparent in both youngsters and young adults; prevalence in the latter group dropped from 25.1% in 1979 to 21.1% in 1982. Current users comprise only a small percentage of those who have ever tried a hallucinogen. Most people have used these drugs on 10 or fewer occasions. Twenty-one percent of those age 18 to 25 years have tried a hallucinogen, but only 1.7% reported using any within the month before the 1982 survey. The lifetime prevalence or ever-used rates of PCP are summarized in Table 4–9. Declines in PCP use are apparent for both youngsters and young adults; prevalence in the latter group dropped from 14.5% in 1979 to 10.5% in 1982 (Table 4–9). It should be remembered that the rates for older adults reflect "ever used" patterns of the 1970s. Although a higher percentage of students age 12 to 17 years before 1976 reported using hallucinogens as they passed from the sixth to the twelfth grade, this trend has been decreasing since 1976 (Figure 4–8).

FIG. 4–7. Trends in use of hallucinogens, 1975–1981

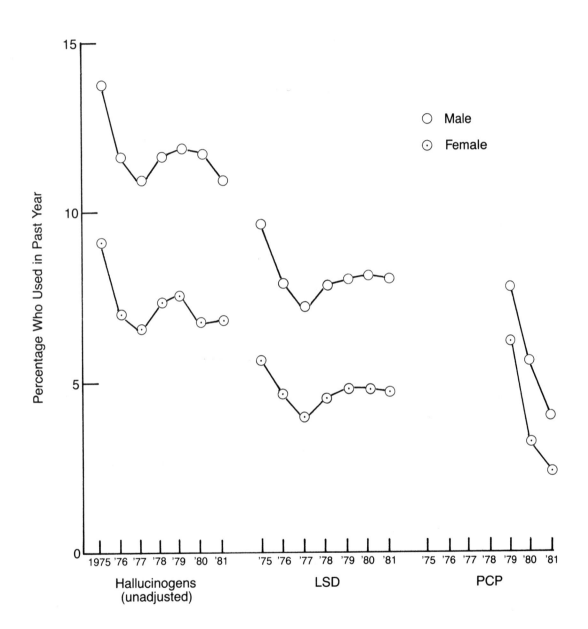

Source: Alcohol, Drug Abuse and Mental Health Administration.

FIG. 4-8.   Hallucinogens: trends in lifetime prevalence for earlier grade levels based on retrospective reports from seniors, 1969–1981

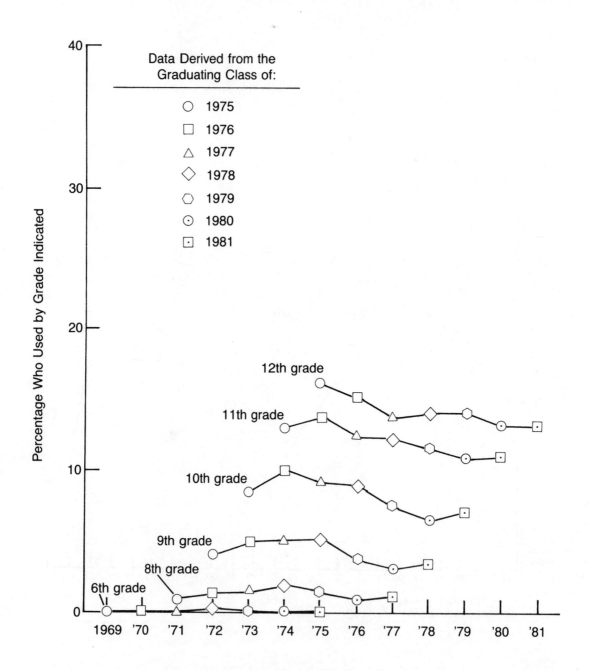

Source: Alcohol, Drug Abuse and Mental Health Administration.

TABLE 4–10. Hallucinogens: Youth, Young Adults, and Older Adults, 1982

PATTERNS	YOUTH (age 12–17 years) (1581)	YOUNG ADULTS (age 18–25 years) (1283)	OLDER ADULTS (age 26+ years) (2760)
Lifetime Frequency of Use:			
1 or 2 times	1.2%	5.0%	1.8%
3 to 10 times	2.0	7.8	2.0
11 to 99 times	0.9	4.4	2.0
100 or more times	*	1.1	*
Not sure how many times	1.0	2.9	*
Never used hallucinogens	94.8	78.9	93.6
Marijuana Use on Same Occasion:			
Nearly every time	2.3%	7.9%	2.0%
About one-half the time	0.6	2.2	.5
Occasionally/rarely	*	4.6	1.8
Never	1.1	3.7	1.6
Not sure if on same occasion	0.8	2.6	0.5
Never used hallucinogens	94.8	78.9	93.6
Current Use:			
Days Used in Past Month:			
20 or more	*	*	*
5–19	*	*	*
3–4	*	*	*
1–2	0.6	1.2	*
Not past month user	3.8	19.4	6.3
Not sure how many days	*	*	*
Never used hallucinogens	94.8	78.9	93.6

Note: Numbers in parenthesis indicate size of sample; some categories do not add to 100% because of rounding
*Less than 0.5%
Source: Alcohol, Drug Abuse and Mental Health Administration

TABLE 4–11. Young Adults 18 to 25 in Various Subgroups Using Hallucinogens Currently, 1977 Survey, and Projections for 1985, 1990, and 1995

SUBGROUPS OF YOUNG ADULTS	1977	1985	1990	1995
Females	228*	223	202	186
Males	495	483	438	406
Whites	586	562	501	456
Nonwhites	92	100	98	97
Large Metropolitan Residents	304	297	269	249
Other Metropolitan Residents	197	193	175	161
Nonmetropolitan Residents	74	170	154	142

*Numbers are in thousands and based on 1977 prevalence rates.
Source: Alcohol, Drug Abuse and Mental Health Administration

Many hallucinogen users report a concomitant use of marijuana on the same occasion. The group who were teenagers during the 1970s reported the greatest use of these drugs (Table 4–10).

The projection of how many persons will be current users of hallucinogenic drugs based on data gathered in the late 1970s is shown in Table 4–11. Significant falls in the use of several of these drugs after the late 1970s portend even lower use than the projected numbers show.

COCAINE

An increasingly popular drug in the 1970s, is cocaine. A white powder obtained from the coca plant that grows along the western slopes of the Andes, it is now being cultivated in other countries. A CNS stimulant, in small doses it produces euphoria and heightens physical strength. In larger amounts, it triggers mental confusion and convulsions.

During the initial phase of its popularity, cocaine advocates represented it as a safe nonaddictive drug. But it is now known to be psychologically addictive. And some persons become physically addicted as well in that they develop withdrawal symptoms. Chronic abuse promotes a tendency to violent and antisocial behavior, personality disturbances, and sleep and appetite disturbances prompting emaciation.

Paranoia is symptomatic of users who develop a toxic psychosis. Deep depression ensues following IV administration. This reaction typically aggravates desire for another dose. Although cocaine can be inhaled, IV absorption is popular in the United States and produces a much stronger predepression reaction. To dilute the excitatory effect of IV use, many addicts mix cocaine with heroin. Other abusers frequently mix cocaine with marijuana. The adverse effects produced by abuse often propel users to experiment with other drugs to sustain the euphoria or wellbeing that they derive only with cocaine or another substitute. In 1986, the danger posed by cocaine use was exacerbated with the introduction of a very pure form that can be synthesized in any home kitchen. Called "crack" in junkie argot, it causes greatly intensified psychophysiologic reactions among addicts. Now widely available, crack has engendered much community concern, media attention, and a stronger resolve among government officials and citizens to counter the drug epidemic through education.

Trends in the lifetime prevalence and recent monthly use of cocaine during the 1970s do not reflect the new use of crack. But these pre-crack data are dismaying in themselves with the lifetime prevalence of cocaine use increasing among 18- to 25-year-olds from 9.1% in 1972 to 27.5% in 1979. This trend tapered off to a 1% increase between 1979 and 1982. Use by older and younger adults has not been as great. Users in the younger and older age groups also report using cocaine only once, where as those between age 18 and 25 years are frequent users.

A breakdown of cocaine users by age, sex, race, education, and residence is presented in Table 4–12. The most common user is a white male college graduate living in the northeast or west in a large metropolitan area, a profile that also fits users of several other drugs.

The actual frequency of cocaine use and the times it is used with marijuana are summarized in Table 4–13. Almost 10% of those between age 18 and 25 years use marijuana every time they use cocaine. Those using cocaine 1 or 2 days in the month before being surveyed were mostly between 18 and 25 years.

Unlike the trend in drug introduction at various grade levels for marijuana and the hallucinogens, the trend for cocaine shows no sign of a decline. The class of 1981 shows the highest percentage of users at every grade level except the sixth and eighth (Figure 4–9). The projection of those who will be cocaine users through 1995 is summarized in Table 4–14.

Several prescription medications can be obtained illegally and used for other purposes. In this category are substances known in the vernacular as "uppers" and "downers." They include amphetamines, which are stimulants, barbiturates or sedatives, and tranquilizers, which unlike sedatives calm the user without modifying the pain response.

TABLE 4–12. Recency of Cocaine Use Among Subgroups of Young Adults, 1982

SUBGROUP	EVER USED (%)	PAST MONTH (%)	PAST YEAR, NOT PAST MONTH (%)	NOT PAST YEAR (%)	NEVER USED (%)
Young Adults (age 18–25 years)	28.3	6.8	11.9	9.5	71.7
Age:					
18–21 years	26	7	11	8	74
22–25 years	31	7	13	11	69
Sex:					
Male	35	9	16	9	65
Female	22	5	8	10	78
Race:					
White	30	7	13	10	70
Black and other races	18	3	7	8	82
Education:					
Non-high school graduate	23	4	11	8	77
High school graduate	28	6	11	11	72
Attended college	31	9	13	9	69
Completed 1–3 years	30	7	13	10	70
Graduate	34	13	14	6	66
Now a full-time college student	29	7	14	8	71
Region:					
Northeast	35	13	12	10	65
North Central	25	3	10	11	75
South	21	4	8	9	79
West	38	9	21	8	62
Population density:					
Large metropolitan	35	10	14	11	65
Small metropolitan	27	6	12	8	73
Nonmetropolitan	22	5	8	9	78

Note: Some categories do not add to 100% because of rounding.
Source: National Institute on Drug Abuse

TABLE 4–13. Cocaine: Youth, Young Adults, and Older Adults, 1982

PATTERN	YOUTH: AGE 12–17 (%)	YOUNG ADULTS: AGE 18–25 (%)	OLDER ADULTS: AGE 26+ (%)
Lifetime frequency of use:			
1 or 2 times	3.7	7.4	2.5
3 to 10 times	1.8	9.2	3.3
11 to 99 times	0.9	9.1	2.3
100 or more times	*	2.5	0.5
Not sure how many times	*	*	*
Never used cocaine	93.5	71.7	91.5
Marijuana use on the same occasion:			
Nearly every time	2.1	9.6	2.8
About one-half the time	0.9	2.7	0.7
Occasionally/rarely	1.3	7.7	2.3
Never	2.2	8.2	2.7
Not sure if on same occasion	*	*	*
Never used cocaine	93.5	71.7	91.5
Current Use:			
Days used in past month:			
20 or more	*	*	*
5–19	0.5	1.3	*
3–4	0.4	1.0	*
1–2	0.7	4.3	0.8
Not past month user	4.8	21.5	7.3
Not sure how many days	*	*	*
Never used cocaine	93.5	71.7	91.5

Note: Some categories do not add to 100% because of rounding.
*Less than 0.5%.
Source: Alcohol, Drug Abuse and Mental Health Administration

TABLE 4–14. Young Adults 18 to 25 in Various Subgroups Using Cocaine Currently, 1977 Survey, and Projections for 1985, 1990, and 1995

SUBGROUPS OF YOUNG ADULTS	1977	1985	1990	1995
Females	260*	254	230	213
Males	973	950	861	798
Whites	977	937	834	759
Nonwhites	261	283	278	277
Large Metropolitan Residents	773	756	685	633
Other Metropolitan Residents	266	260	236	218
Nonmetropolitan Residents	153	150	136	125

*Numbers are in thousands and based on 1977 prevalence rates.
Source: Alcohol, Drug Abuse and Mental Health Administration

FIG. 4–9.   Cocaine: trends in lifetime prevalence for earlier grade levels based on retrospective reports from seniors, 1969–1981

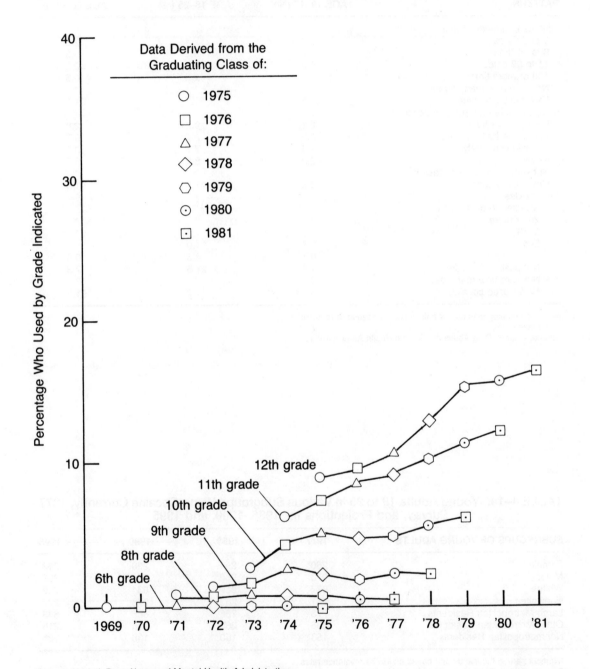

Source: Alcohol, Drug Abuse and Mental Health Administration.

AMPHETAMINES

Amphetamines include well-known stimulants, such as Benzedrine, Dexedrine, and methamphetamine, or Methedrine. They are used legally and illegally, to relieve depression, fatigue, pregnancy-related nausea, and obesity. Their abuse stems from their use as mood-altering drugs. Amphetamine abusers take them with barbiturates and alcohol to achieve mood elevation.

The dangers of amphetamine are multiple. Those unused to them, e.g., who have no tolerance, may develop a psychotic reaction with hallucinations and paranoid delusions by taking a single dose of no more than 50 mg. The lethal dose is about 900 mg, but users who have developed a tolerance take daily doses as large as 1g. Usually, amphetamines are taken orally. Chronic users, however, who develop high tolerance often take them intravenously as "speed." Those who take amphetamines by this route have a high incidence of serum hepatitis as do other IV drug abusers.

The psychosis-producing penchant of amphetamines was noted in 1939 when these drugs were first developed. Of all the drugs that are abused, including LSD, amphetamine psychosis most closely mimics schizophrenia. Suicide is not an uncommon result of chronic amphetamine abuse; those in drug-induced psychosis are often treated with antischizophrenic drugs. Other effects include apathy and loss of initiative lasting for months after discontinuation. Although withdrawal symptoms do not develop, the blasé feeling that develops when amphetamine ingestion is discontinued often prompts resumption of use.

Amphetamine adverse effects include hypertension, increased heart rate, and sometimes muscle tremor and twitching. Study of long-term methamphetamine users has uncovered organic brain damage as well.

BARBITURATES

Barbiturates are similar to but not as potent as anesthetics. They induce relaxation and mild euphoria. Although at low levels they do not usually cause drowsiness, there may be some functional impairment. At higher doses, barbiturates induce sleep and can cause several undesirable effects, such as nausea, delirium, mental confusion, and diarrhea. Depending on dose, sleep can be so deep that the user cannot be awakened and may suffer respiratory depression and shock leading to death. Signs physicians look for in the chronic barbiturate user are slowed thought, slurring of speech, and bruises on the extremities since users often fall.

Psychological dependence can develop, but physical dependence, which is evident in withdrawal, does develop with doses in the 100- to 200-mg range. In higher concentration, discontinuance can trigger withdrawal symptoms more severe than those associated with opiates (narcotics). Barbiturates should never be withdrawn suddenly from the long-time user; detoxification often takes place in a hospital setting because of the extreme danger it can pose. The ultimate effects of chronic use approximate many of the symptoms of the alcoholic, namely blackouts, slurred speech, poor motor coordination, mood swings, and psychosis.

TRANQUILIZERS

Tranquilizers reduce anxiety and nervousness. They were popularized in the mid-20th century by psychiatrists when they noticed that reserpine and chlorpromazine had calming effects. Because reserpine also caused depression, ulcers, low blood pressure, and weakness, chlorpromazine and other more recently synthesized tranquilizers have replaced it. These drugs are used widely and have been particularly prescribed for women whose physical complaints have often been ascribed to "nervousness" by physicians. The phenothiazines may produce jaundice, dermatitis, and convulsions. Other milder tranquilizers, such as Miltown and Equanil, are considered to be safe without adverse side effects. But heavy, prolonged use can result in physical dependence, which elicits severe withdrawal symptoms, such as insomnia, hallucination, convulsions, and tremors.

These psychotherapeutic drugs require a doctor's prescription. But they are also used nonmedically primarily by persons age 18 to 25 years (Table 4–15). Smaller numbers of people older and younger have tried them, too (Tables 4–16 and 4–17). Illicit use among the high-risk age group is primarily of sedatives and stimulants; prescription abuse, on the other hand, is associated more with tranquilizers. The reason for this may, of course, be that tranquilizers, which are readily prescribed by doctors, are available. Hence, those who want them do not have to obtain them through illicit channels. In contrast, physicians are more reluctant to prescribe barbiturates and amphetamines. The trend in recency of use among young adults age 18 to 25 years is shown in Table 4–15.

Among older adults, the recency of use according to several characteristics of this population group is presented in Table 4–16. The usage pattern indicates higher usage in the west, among those who have attended or graduated from college, and among males. Use among both races is about equal.

TABLE 4–15. Nonmedical Use: Recency of Nonmedical Use of Any Psychotherapeutic Drug Among Subgroups of Young Adults, 1982

SUBGROUP	EVER USED (%)	PAST MONTH (%)	PAST YEAR, NOT PAST MONTH (%)	NOT PAST YEAR (%)	NEVER USED (%)
Young adults (age 18–25 years):	28.4	7.0	9.1	12.3	71.6
Age:					
18–21	27	8	9	11	73
22–25	29	7	9	13	71
Sex:					
Male	33	8	11	14	67
Female	24	6	8	11	76
Race:					
White	31	8	10	13	69
Black and other races	14	4	4	6	86
Education:					
Non-high school graduate	28	8	11	9	72
High school graduate	27	7	9	12	73
Attended college:	29	7	8	14	71
Completed 1–3 years	29	8	9	12	71
Graduate	30	5	6	18	70
Now a full-time college student	26	6	9	11	74
Region:					
Northeast	28	4	8	15	72
North Central	30	11	9	10	70
South	28	7	9	12	72
West	28	5	9	14	72
Population density:					
Large metropolitan	32	6	10	16	68
Small metropolitan	26	6	9	10	74
Nonmetropolitan	28	10	8	11	72

Note: Some categories do not add to 100% because of rounding.
Source: Alcohol, Drug Abuse and Mental Health Administration

TABLE 4–16. Nonmedical Use: Recency of Nonmedical Use of Any Psychotherapeutic Drug Among Subgroups of Older Adults, 1982

SUBGROUP	EVER USED (%)	PAST MONTH (%)	PAST YEAR, NOT PAST MONTH (%)	NOT PAST YEAR (%)	NEVER USED (%)
Older Adults (age 26+ years):	8.8	1.2	1.8	5.7	91.2
Age (in years):					
26–29	25	5	5	14	75
30–34	18	4	5	10	82
35–49	11	*	2	9	89
50+	1	*	*	1	99
Sex:					
Male	12	2	3	8	88
Female	6	1	1	4	94
Race:					
White	9	1	2	6	91
Black and other races	8	1	3	4	92
Education:					
Non-high school graduate	3	*	1	2	97
High school graduate	7	2	1	4	93
Attended college:	15	2	3	11	85
Completed 1–3 years	11	1	4	7	89
Graduate	19	2	2	14	81
Region:					
Northeast	9	1	1	6	91
North Central	8	2	2	4	92
South	6	1	1	4	94
West	14	1	3	9	86
Population density:					
Large metropolitan	10	1	2	7	90
Small metropolitan	9	2	2	5	91
Nonmetropolitan	6	1	1	4	94

Note: Some categories do not add to 100% because of rounding.
*Less than 0.5%
Source: Alcohol, Drug Abuse and Mental Health Administration

Among subgroups of youngsters, females are slightly greater users of some psychotherapeutic drugs as are whites. Users are fairly evenly distributed throughout the United States, with a higher prevalence in the northeast for stimulants or sedatives (Table 4–17). Data for those ever having any experience with these drugs even once are presented by age group in Table 4–18. The introduction of sedatives, barbiturates, and tranquilizers to youngsters and children declined in the late 1970s after peaking at each grade level in the mid-1970s. However, since 1979, there seems to be a slight upturn again in the percentage of youngsters who try these drugs at early grade levels through high school. The trends for each of these types of drug are shown in Figures 4–10 to 4–12.

Although the data for sedatives, barbiturates, and tranquilizers show a recent upsurge, they are more encouraging by far than those for stimulants and amphetamines (Figure 4–13). Thirty-four percent of the class of 1981 indicated exposure to these stimulants. Five percent had used them by the ninth grade.

Analysts believe that the drastic increase in amphetamine use represents increased availability of over-the-counter preparations that are milder than former agents, but this is difficult to determine.

One clear determinate of increased drug use is knowledge of the drug's effects. If one considers the current increased use of amphetamines, one finds correlated with it a decreased perception of its danger. Despite the fact that these drugs produce severe psychosis, the perceived danger is less among young people in the early 1980s than it was in the 1970s. An increased awareness for most other drugs corresponds with declines in their use (Table 4–19).

Social disapproval of a drug also ties in with the prevalence of its use (Table 4–20). Once again, disapproval of amphetamine use is less severe in recent years probably because of the mistaken notion that they are not harmful.

Another correlation of drug use is availability. Except for hallucinogens and heroin, the perceived availability of most drugs—particularly amphetamines and barbiturates—has risen (Figure 4–14). While the perceived availability of barbiturates jumped 6%, there was no corresponding increase in their use. The jump of 8% for amphetamines was again attended by an increase in use.

Additional understanding of the extent of drug use can be determined from data on the senior high school class of 1981. As Figure 4–15 shows, the most popular substances were alcohol, nicotine, marijuana, stimulants, and cocaine.

The age at which people entered federally funded drug treatment programs in 1978 is depicted in Table 4–21. The trend in treatment loads in centers for drug abuse excluding alcohol treatment from

TABLE 4-17. Nonmedical Use: Nonmedical Experience with Types of Psychotherapeutic Drugs Among Subgroups of Youth, 1982

SUBGROUP	EVER USED				
	Stimulants (%)	Sedatives (%)	Tranquilizers (%)	Analgesics (%)	Any Psychotherapeutic (%)
Youth (age 12–17 years)	6.7	5.8	4.9	4.2	10.3
Age (in years):					
12–13	2	3	1	2	4
14–15	4	4	3	2	7
16–17	13	10	10	8	19
Sex:					
Male	6	6	6	5	9
Female	7	6	4	4	11
Race:					
White	7	7	5	5	11
Black and other races	3	1	2	2	5
Region:					
Northeast	8	7	4	3	13
North Central	7	5	7	4	10
South	7	6	6	5	9
West	5	5	2	4	10
Population density:					
Large metropolitan	7	7	6	5	11
Small metropolitan	7	5	5	5	10
Nonmetropolitan	5	6	4	3	10

Source: Alcohol, Drug Abuse and Mental Health Administration

TABLE 4–18. Nonmedical Experience with Types of Psychotherapeutic Drugs Among Youth, Young Adults, and Older Adults, 1972–1982

DRUG TYPE	EVER USED					
	1972 (%)	1974 (%)	1976 (%)	1977 (%)	1979 (%)	1982 (%)
Stimulants:						
Youth	4	5	4.4	5.2	3.4	6.7
Young adults	12	17	16.6	21.2	18.2	18.0
Older adults	3	3	5.6	4.7	5.8	6.2
Sedatives:						
Youth	3	5	2.8	3.1	3.2	5.8
Young adults	10	15	11.9	18.4	17.0	18.7
Older adults	2	2	2.4	2.8	3.5	4.8
Tranquilizers:						
Youth	3	3	3.3	3.8	4.1	4.9
Young adults	7	10	9.1	13.4	15.8	15.1
Older adults	5	2	2.7	2.6	3.1	3.6
Analgesics:						
Youth	X	X	X	X	3.2	4.2
Young adults	X	X	X	X	11.8	12.1
Older adults	X	X	X	X	2.7	3.2

Note: an "X" indicates that data is not available.
Source: Alcohol, Drug Abuse and Mental Health Administration

FIG. 4–10.   Sedatives: trends in lifetime prevalence for earlier grade levels based on retrospective reports from seniors, 1969–1981

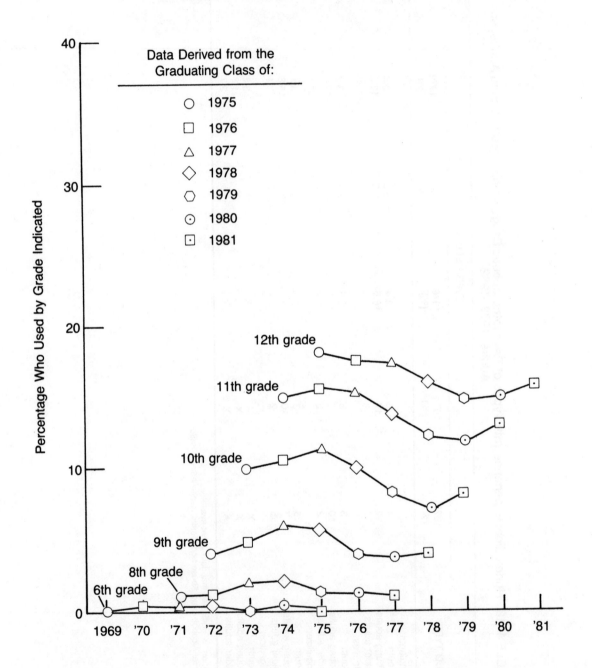

Source: Alcohol, Drug Abuse and Mental Health Administration.

FIG. 4–11.   Barbiturates: trends in lifetime prevalence for earlier grade levels based on retrospective reports from seniors, 1969–1981

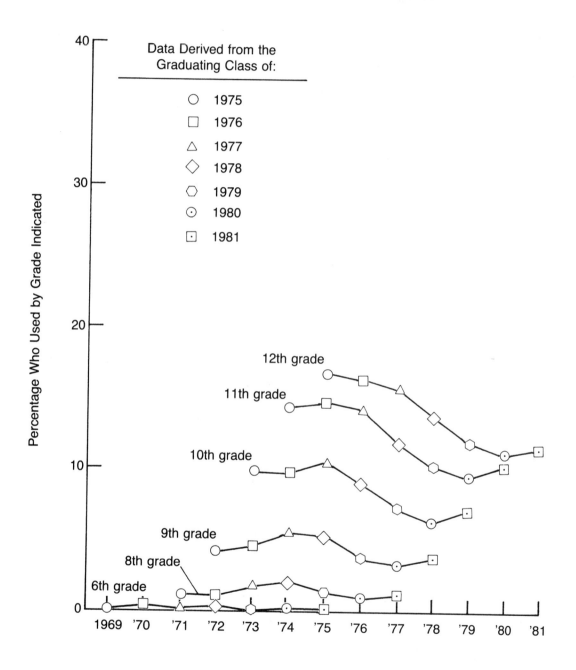

Source: Alcohol, Drug Abuse and Mental Health Administration.

FIG. 4–12.   Tranquilizers: trends in lifetime prevalence for earlier grade levels based on retrospective reports from seniors, 1969–1981

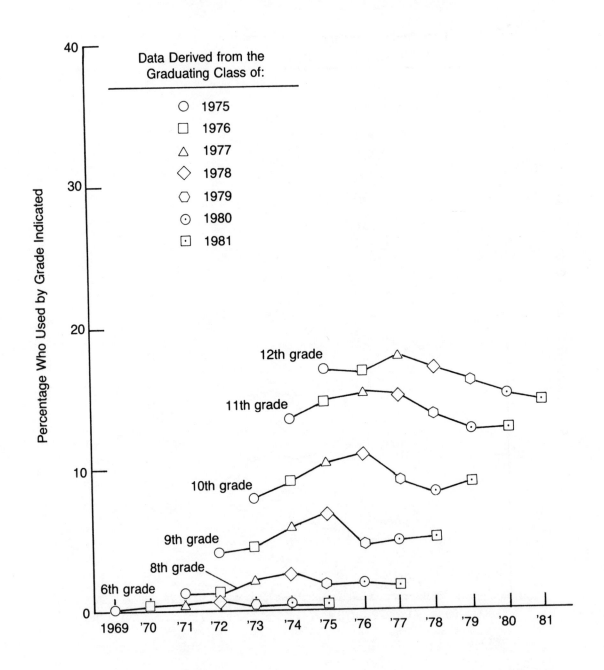

Source: Alcohol, Drug Abuse and Mental Health Administration.

FIG. 4–13. Stimulants: trends in lifetime prevalence for earlier grade levels based on retrospective reports from seniors, 1969–1981

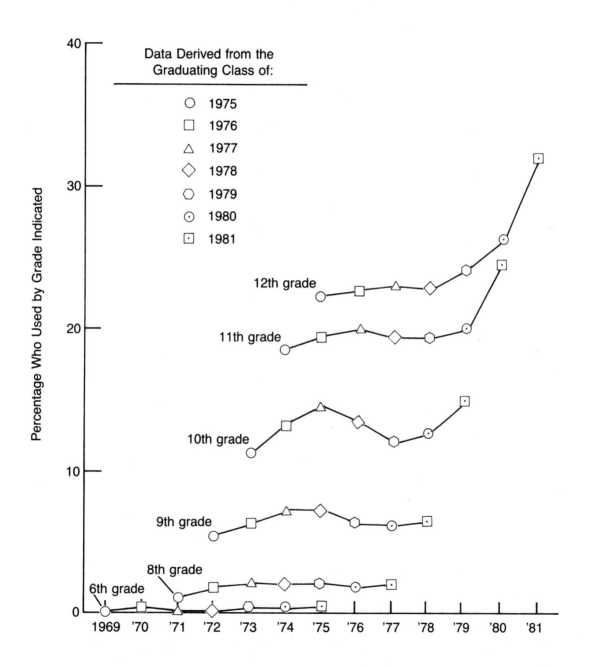

Source: Alcohol, Drug Abuse and Mental Health Administration.

TABLE 4–19. Trends in Perceived Harmfulness of Drugs, 1975–1981

Q. HOW MUCH DO YOU THINK PEOPLE RISK HARMING THEMSELVES PHYSICALLY OR IN OTHER WAYS IF THEY . . .	PERCENTAGE SAYING "GREAT RISK"*							
	Class of 1975	Class of 1976	Class of 1977	Class of 1978	Class of 1979	Class of 1980	Class of 1981	'80–'81 change
Try marijuana once or twice	15.1	11.4	9.5	8.1	9.4	10.0	13.0	+3.0ss
Smoke marijuana occasionally	18.1	15.0	13.4	12.4	13.5	14.7	19.1	+4.4sss
Smoke marijuana regularly	43.3	38.6	36.4	34.9	42.0	50.4	57.6	+7.2sss
Try LSD once or twice	49.4	45.7	43.2	42.7	41.6	43.9	45.5	+1.6
Take LSD regularly	81.4	80.8	79.1	81.1	82.4	83.0	83.5	+0.5
Try cocaine once or twice	42.6	39.1	35.6	33.2	31.5	31.3	32.1	+0.8
Take cocaine regularly	73.1	72.3	68.2	68.2	69.5	69.2	71.2	+2.0
Try heroin once or twice	60.1	58.9	55.8	52.9	50.4	52.1	52.9	-0.1
Take heroin occasionally	75.6	75.6	71.9	71.4	70.9	70.9	72.2	+1.3
Take heroin regularly	87.2	88.6	86.1	86.6	87.5	86.2	87.5	+1.3
Try amphetamines once or twice	35.4	33.4	30.8	29.9	29.7	29.7	26.4	-3.3s
Take amphetamines regularly	69.0	67.3	66.6	67.1	69.9	69.1	66.1	-3.0s
Try a barbiturate once or twice	34.8	32.5	31.2	31.3	30.7	30.9	28.4	-2.5
Take barbiturates regularly	69.1	67.7	68.6	68.4	71.6	72.2	69.9	-2.3
Try one or two drinks of an alcoholic beverage (beer, wine, liquor)	5.3	4.8	4.1	3.4	4.1	3.8	4.6	+0.8
Take one or two drinks nearly every day	21.5	21.2	18.5	19.6	22.6	20.3	21.6	+1.3
Take four or five drinks nearly every day	63.5	61.0	62.9	63.1	66.2	65.7	64.5	-1.2
Have five or more drinks once or twice each weekend	37.8	37.0	34.7	34.5	34.9	35.9	36.3	+0.4
Smoke one or more packs of cigarettes daily	51.3	56.4	58.4	59.0	63.0	63.7	63.3	-0.4
N =	(2804)	(3225)	(3570)	(3770)	(3250)	(3234)	(3604)	

Note: Level of significance of difference between the two most recent classes: s=0.05, ss=0.01, sss=0.001.
*Answer alternatives were: (1) No risk, (2) Slight risk, (3) Moderate risk, (4) Great risk, and (5) Can't say, Drug unfamiliar
Source: Alcohol, Drug Abuse and Mental Health Administration

TABLE 4-20. Trends in Proportions Disapproving of Drug Use, 1975–1981

Q. DO YOU DISAPPROVE OF PEOPLE (WHO ARE 18 OR OLDER) DOING EACH OF THE FOLLOWING?†	PERCENTAGE "DISAPPROVING"*							
	Class of 1975	Class of 1976	Class of 1977	Class of 1978	Class of 1979	Class of 1980	Class of 1981	'80–'81 change
Try marijuana once or twice	47.0	38.4	33.4	33.4	34.2	39.0	40.0	+1.0
Smoke marijuana occasionally	54.8	47.8	44.3	43.5	45.3	49.7	52.6	+2.9
Smoke marijuana regularly	71.9	69.5	65.5	67.5	69.2	74.6	77.4	+2.8s
Try LSD once or twice	82.8	84.6	83.9	85.4	86.6	87.3	86.4	−0.9
Take LSD regularly	94.1	95.3	95.8	96.4	96.9	96.7	96.8	+0.1
Try cocaine once or twice	81.3	82.4	79.1	77.0	74.7	76.3	74.6	−1.7
Take cocaine regularly	93.3	93.9	92.1	91.9	90.8	91.1	90.7	−0.4
Try heroin once or twice	91.5	92.6	92.5	92.0	93.4	93.5	93.5	0.0
Take heroin occasionally	94.8	96.0	96.0	96.4	96.8	96.7	97.2	+0.5
Take heroin regularly	96.7	97.5	97.2	97.8	97.9	97.6	97.8	+0.2
Try amphetamines once or twice	74.8	75.1	74.2	74.8	75.1	75.4	71.1	−4.3ss
Take amphetamines regularly	92.1	92.8	92.5	93.5	94.4	93.0	91.7	−1.3
Try barbiturates once or twice	77.7	81.3	81.1	82.4	84.0	83.9	82.4	−1.5
Take barbiturates regularly	93.3	93.6	93.0	94.3	95.2	95.4	94.2	−1.2
Try one or two drinks of an alcoholic beverage (beer, wine, liquor)	21.6	18.2	15.6	15.6	15.8	16.0	17.2	+1.2
Take one or two drinks nearly every day	67.6	68.9	66.8	67.7	68.3	69.0	69.1	+0.1
Take four or five drinks nearly every day	88.7	90.7	88.4	90.2	91.7	90.8	91.8	+1.0
Have five or more drinks once or twice each weekend	60.3	58.6	57.4	56.2	56.7	55.6	55.5	−0.1
Smoke one or more packs of cigarettes daily	67.5	65.9	66.4	67.0	70.3	70.8	69.9	−0.9
N =	(2677)	(3234)	(3582)	(3686)	(3221)	(3261)	(3610)	

Note: Level of significance of difference between the two most recent classes: s=0.05, ss=0.01, sss=0.001.
*Answer alternatives were: (1) Don't disapprove, (2) Disapprove, and (3) Strongly disapprove.
Percentages are shown for categories (2) and (3) combined.
†The 1975 question asked about people who are "20 or older."

FIG. 4-14. Trends in perceived availability of drugs, 1975-1981

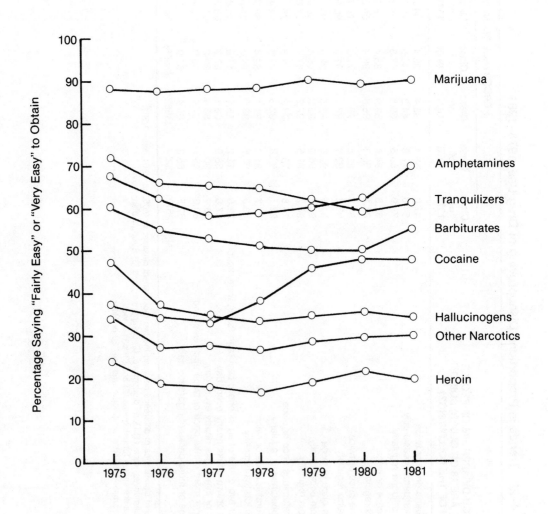

Source: Alcohol, Drug Abuse and Mental Health Administration.

FIG. 4–15. Prevalence and recency of use for 11 types of drugs, class of 1981

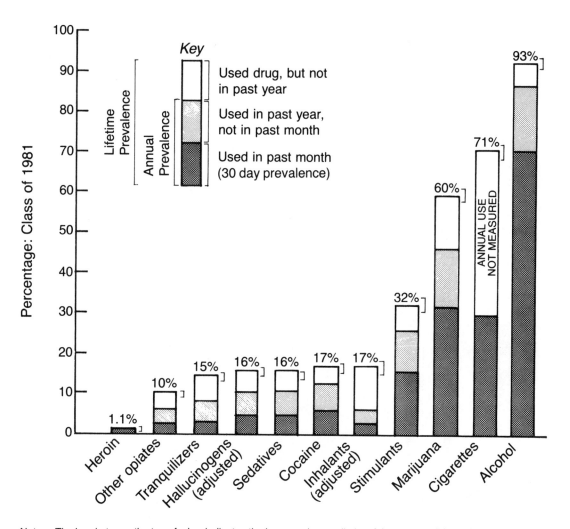

Note: The bracket near the top of a bar indicates the lower and upper limits of the 95% confidence interval.

Source: Alcohol, Drug Abuse and Mental Health Administration.

TABLE 4–21. Age at Time of Admission to Federally Funded Drug Treatment Programs, 1978 (regional drug situation analysis)

AGE (years)	NATIONWIDE (%)	NORTHEASTERN REGION Phila. SMSA (%)	NORTH CENTRAL REGION Chicago SMSA (%)	SOUTHEASTERN REGION Miami SMSA (%)	SOUTH CENTRAL REGION Dallas SMSA (%)	WESTERN REGION Los Angeles SMSA (%)
Under 18	11.4	8.4	5.8	21.2	5.5	5.0
18–25	38.2	38.3	34.5	39.5	39.5	36.0
26–44	45.1	49.0	55.4	35.3	50.1	52.8
44+	5.2	4.4	4.3	4.0	5.0	6.3

Source: Alcohol, Drug Abuse and Mental Health Administration

1977 to 1982 are shown in Table 4–22. The admissions to treatment centers by drug used are displayed in Table 4–23. Between 1975 and 1979, admissions for almost every popular drug rose dramatically. Heroin admissions were down, but other opiate admissions rose steeply in 1979 vs 1975.

The interplay of mental disease, drug abuse, and suicide is evident from the welter of data discussed in this volume. Each of the factors scrutinized is involved in the rising tide of adolescent and young adult death vis-à-vis homicide, drug overdose, and suicide.

TABLE 4–22. Drug Abuse Treatment Units: 1977–1982 [In thousands, except as noted. 1977 as of April 30; 1980 and 1982 as of Sept. 30. Includes Puerto Rico, Guam, and the Virgin Islands. Treatment unit refers to a facility that specifically provides direct, on-site drug abuse treatment services to its clients. Based on a complete census of all known units; for 1982, the response rate was 89.4%]

ITEM	1977	1980	1982	ITEM	1977	1980	1982
Treatment units (number)	3,147	3,449	3,018	Clients			
				Outpatient and day care	203.3	157.2	149.5
Clients*	234.6	181.5	196.3	Residential	18.5	15.1	14.8
				Hospital inpatient	3.7	2.6	2.9
By mode of treatment:				Prison	9.1	6.6	6.2
Drug free†	147.2	105.0	95.9				
Detoxification‡	5.8	5.2	5.1	Total funding (mil. dol.)	510.7	486.6	533.6
Methadone maintenance**	80.0	67.9	72.0	Total staff	40.5	36.0¶	34.0¶

*Includes items not shown separately.
†Drug withdrawal without medication.
‡Drug withdrawal supported by use of prescribed medication. If methadone used, treatment for 21 days or less.
**Continued use of methadone for a period of more than 21 days. Includes other maintenance treatments.
¶Includes staff for alcoholism treatment when drug abuse and alcoholism are treated at same unit. Full-time equivalent employment.
Source: U.S. National Institute on Drug Abuse, *NIDA Statistical Series*, series F, periodic.

TABLE 4–23. Admissions to Treatment, 1975–1979, United States

DRUG TYPE	1975	1976	1977	1978	1979
Heroin	116,948	137,678	111,289	100,131	95,198
Methadone	1,512	1,302	2,626	3,735	3,105
Other opiates	4,513	4,736	7,190	11,098	14,481
Marijuana	30,695	20,751	21,141	30,074	38,222
Barbiturates	10,180	10,524	10,068	10,144	9,213
Amphetamines	9,242	10,376	10,526	13,355	15,370
Hallucinogens (including PCP)	5,526	5,484	7,610	11,637	14,807
Cocaine	2,192	2,777	3,610	5,902	9,028
Tranquilizers and other sedatives	4,638	6,358	8,235	10,696	12,746
Inhalants	2,380	2,742	2,898	3,323	3,373
Over-the-counter drugs	386	437	469	668	598

Source: Alcohol, Drug Abuse and Mental Health Administration

A Note On Methodology

This volume and the others in this series are concerned with the demographics of disease, and the disease patterns of different groups of people considered on the basis of age, sex, or cultural grouping. The study of these patterns and the causes of disease in large and small populations is called *epidemiology.*

For thousands of years, people believed that sickness was a punishment for transgressions against the gods. The pattern of sinfulness followed by sickness was evident often enough, for people seldom lived perfect lives and seldom avoided all disease. When sick, they would call for a shaman, a priest-doctor who would beg the gods through prayer and incantation to restore the sick to health.

As simplistic as this approach seems to many modern peoples, the basic impetus of early peoples was epidemiologic. They had isolated a pattern of disease and sought to avoid the scourge of disease by addressing its cause, an angry god.

Gradually, exceptions to the accepted pattern of disease were noticed. Epidemics affected virtually everyone in a community, good or bad. So, too, people began to notice other patterns of illness and linked aspects of their natural surroundings, such as their drinking water and certain foods, to the development of disease.

People also noticed that those in contact with a sick person often developed the same symptoms a few days or weeks later. Thus, a belief developed that disease could be transmitted somehow from person to person, perhaps by the movement of invisible particles traveling from the body of the sick person to that of the well one. The writings of Lucretius described this theory of contagious disease. With this pattern of disease noticed, the stage was set for the development of modern epidemiology, the science that looks for the pattern of diseases and the natural causes evidenced by that pattern.

Although the stage was set, many obstacles still had to be overcome. Autopsy examinations were forbidden through most of the Middle Ages, and everyday observational tools used by the modern physician, such as the clinical thermometer and the stethoscope, were not invented until the 17th and 18th centuries, respectively. Thus, it was difficult to diagnose the cause of death in many instances. Those who hazarded a guess were often wildly simplistic or incorrect.

Even in the 20th century, influenza, pneumonia, bronchitis, and tuberculosis have routinely been mistaken for each other. Autopsies performed in the latter part of this century finally helped to clarify mortality from this cause.

THE DEATH CERTIFICATE

Despite today's much improved knowledge of the body and disease, the problems of relying on the information entered on a death certificate are notorious. Unfortunately, mortality data reported by countries around the world are based of necessity on death-certificate entries.

In many countries, death-certificate entries represent a physician's diagnosis. But in many other countries, the cause of death is reported by the deceased's relatives to a local clerk. Even in more sophisticated countries, listing the cause of death often obscures the real pathologic profile. For example, dying is always a dualistic event resulting from the interaction of a given host and the disease agent that afflicts the host. In one person, influenza may prove fatal because he is constitutionally weak, perhaps from age or other diseases. In another person, encounter with the influenza virus would be a minor event—in no way life threatening. But the record of influenza mortality translates simply into the ferocity or danger of influenza as a disease.

The decline in measles mortality throughout much of the 20th century is another example of the confluence of several factors. Until the recent development of the measles vaccine, nothing had changed in the incidence or severity of measles. But mortality in those stricken with pneumonia, a common fatal sequel of measles, was being reduced by sulfa drugs.

Similarly, much information and understanding are lost insofar as death certificates require a listing of only one cause of death, although secondary causes can be listed on the back. Conventions have been established that priority should be given to the cause that is most often fatal, communicable or acute. But such conventions vary from country to country.

This practice becomes increasingly problematic as populations experience greater longevity, since old people often suffer from several conditions by the time they die of any one cited cause. Someone with diabetes, poor renal function, and congestive heart failure (CHF) is taxed by a cold that develops into acute bronchitis. Medication places an added burden on their kidneys. Difficulty in breathing places an extra oxygen demand on their heart, while their blood sugar is difficult to control. After a few days, their kidneys fail as does their heart and they die. Did the cold kill them? Did the bronchitis? Or was the cause of death heart failure, kidney failure, or diabetes? The physician must make a choice. In England and Wales, the death rate from bronchitis is higher than in most other countries. But these UK countries are inclined to list cases like the one described as a bronchitis death whereas other countries tend to list it as a cardiovascular death.

When a death certificate was introduced in England that asked the physician to list death "as consequence of," the number of deaths ascribed to bronchitis doubled. Deaths from nephritis in Canada and the United States doubled as well, while one-third to one-half of the deaths typically attributed to diabetes were counted for some other cause.

DIFFICULTIES OF NOMENCLATURE AND CLASSIFICATION

Beyond these difficulties are ones of nomenclature and classification. To solve these problems, an International Classification of Diseases has been established, which has been revised from time to time. The current code represents the ninth such revision. But in its attempt to standardize diagnosis from country to country, the classification has posed other problems. As knowledge of diseases has increased, the classification has gradually changed from anatomic groupings to etiologic ones. Rheumatic fever is still listed anatomically as a heart disease because it affects the heart. But if it were true to the trend, it would be listed according to cause and would be regarded as an infectious disease because we now know that rheumatic fever is caused by a bacterium and is infectious. In the fourth revision, brain tumors were removed from the category of nervous system diseases and put with neoplasms, as we realized that these tumors are the results of cancerous growth. During the fourth revision of the code, a more mysterious change was the removal of criminal abortion from accidental death to complication of pregnancy.

Over the years, as diagnosis has become more specific, deaths due to ill-defined causes have also decreased and other heretofore ill-defined diseases, such as various neoplasms, show increased mortality. As populations have aged and physicians have become accustomed to diagnosing the cause of death in the old, several degenerative diseases, such as diabetes, nephritis, ulcer, and cirrhosis, have left the ill-defined category.

CENSUS PROBLEMS

In addition to classification and nomenclature complexities, elementary census biases enter the picture when countries try to calculate their mortality and morbidity rate due to different diseases. These rates are usually expressed as the number of deaths or disease cases per 100,000 population. Sometimes the rates are calculated for men and women separately or for people in different age groups separately. But census numbers are known for their underestimates of population even in advanced countries like the United States. Young children and transient males who travel for their work are often missed in population counts. The 1960 United States census missed an estimated three million people, particularly blacks. Latin Americans tend to report more 5- to 9-year-old children than 0- to 4-year-olds.

Often, information on sex is missing and when asked for their age, people tend to say they are 18 or 21 when these are the ages of majority in a country and 65 when social benefits are available to 65-year-olds. Many people between age 21 and 40 years tend to lower their age when asked. On the other hand, those who do report their true age tend to round their age, especially to even numbers or to ages divisible by five. To compensate for this tendency, researchers often use age intervals when these statistics are compiled.

SURVEYS

Data on morbidity pose yet different problems in that they are usually obtained from health department reports, review of hospital records, or sample surveys of the population. In the United States, physicians are legally obligated to report a large array of diseases, particularly infectious ones, to their health departments. The latter in turn report their data to the Atlanta Centers for Disease Control. Reports come from all of the states, but data gathered independently tend to reveal an under-reporting of disease to the Centers in many instances.

Sometimes hospital records are used for gathering data but these records are often incomplete or have incorrect entries. In addition, hospitalized patients may not reflect the typical patient with a given disease because hospitalized patients are likely to be those who are more severely ill with a specific disease or those who are intractable to less extreme forms of outpatient treatments.

Sample surveys are also subject to misleading findings, depending on how the sample is chosen and how the survey questions are constructed and asked. Data from several large government surveys have been included in this volume. Elaborate statistical sampling methods have been employed to ensure that the surveys are representative. But the questions sometimes fail to elicit pertinent and interesting information. One example can be found in the discussion in *Cardiovascular Disease* that deals with cerebrovascular disease.

A sample of people were asked about their limitation of normal activity due, presumably, to illness. Some were people who had suffered a stroke; others had not. The stroke victims generally showed greater limitation of activity. But these same people were also generally older and perhaps infirm because of other health conditions. There was no indication that their limitation of activity was specifically related to their stroke event. Thus, we do not know, in light of this particular study, how much dysfunction is caused by stroke in the general population compared to other disability conditions of able-bodied people.

The operations and procedures, together with hospital utilization and physician office visits for people with various diagnoses discussed in this work, were obtained from large government studies, such as the National Ambulatory Care Survey and the National Hospital Discharge Survey, which are conducted annually or periodically. Again the focus of these surveys is not always constant from one to another. Comparison of data from an early survey, such as the NHANES I Nutrition Survey with data on some variables measured by a later survey, such as the NHANES II Survey, is not always possible.

RANDOM VARIABILITY

The perspicacious reader must also realize that health data gathered through survey studies are always subject to a certain amount of random variability. More than a century ago, scientists found to their chagrin that whenever any entity is measured multiple times, the measurement varies. This is true even when the measurement is taken by the same person each time using the same instrument in the same way.

In astronomy, this variability came to be known as the personal equation. But this same kind of variability occurs when one obtains data from a random sample presumably representative of a population of interest. Another random sample surveyed in the same way and equally representative typically yields slightly different results. This variability is called the standard error of a particular study.

The importance of keeping in mind that every sample surveyed has a standard error comes into play when comparisons of data expressed as averages are made. Luckily, the standard error of studies is often small; hence, fairly large differences among groups can be accepted as true differences in reality and not merely the reflection of sampling variability.

When reported differences are small, however, one should not conclude that there is in fact a real difference between two groups unless one knows that the standard error of the study samples is smaller than the small reported difference. For a more detailed explanation of sampling variability, see my article, "Randomization and optimal design," *Journal of Chronic Diseases* 36:606–609, 1983.

CRUDE AND AGE-ADJUSTED DATA

Another factor that good health surveys take into account is the age of the groups compared. Clearly, if the blacks interviewed in a study sample were on average 10 years younger than white subjects, one would be mistaken to conclude that whites smoke more than blacks. Obviously, members of groups that smoke to the same degree will show one smoking longer than the other if the members of one group are older than those of the other. The way to correct for age differences when age is likely to affect whether one has an illness or has followed a particular pattern for some time is to compare age-adjusted samples. You will note throughout this volume that crude rates are given as are age-adjusted rates when they are relevant and available.

Since the rates of mortality and morbidity vary among people of different ages, sex, races, and sometimes ethnic and religious backgrounds—particularly in the United States—one has to be mindful of differences in these groups that may account for their differing disease rates. Age is clearly one of these differences that needs to be adjusted for when comparing data. The average and median ages of the black United States population are considerably lower than the white population. Thus, we would expect to see a lower rate of old-age degenerative disease among blacks than among whites when there is no age adjustment. When age is adjusted for or the rate at the same age is compared, epidemiologists have discovered that blacks actually have a higher rate of hypertension than whites.

Another factor not as easily corrected for is access to and utilization of medical resources. If a particular group, such as blacks, are economically less able or socially less inclined to seek medical care when sick, they may ultimately reflect a higher mortality rate from their diseases or a greater morbidity rate as their untreated conditions grow more severe. The higher mortality in such situations should not be regarded as an indication that the higher mortality group has the disease to a greater extent. In other words, blacks may not have more cancer than whites, but they may have a higher cancer mortality rate because they do not receive an early diagnosis or follow treatment regimens for economic or social reasons.

Some researchers speculate that males have a higher general mortality rate than females in part because they tend to seek less medical help for their ailments and fail to follow prescribed treatment regimens for psychological reasons or because it is not convenient for them to see a physician due to career demands.

Aside from the differences in the groups just discussed, differences also exist in groups that may explain why disease does indeed occur more often in some groups than in others. In fact, this is the basic logic of epidemiology and the real incentive for keeping track of vital statistics. Epidemiologists seek to isolate patterns in disease to determine possible pathologic causes.

TELLING PATTERNS

Once it is determined that members of one group are sick and those of another are not, epidemiologists study factors that may be affecting the groups differently. One of the earliest of these investigations was conducted by the physician John Snow, who investigated cholera in London between 1848 and 1854. At that time, different parts of London were supplied with water by different companies. Snow noticed that the cholera cases were confined to areas supplied by two specific water companies. In contrast to the others these two obtained their water from a very polluted section of the Thames River.

One of the companies changed its source farther upriver and when water pipes were laid in the city, its pipes were alternated with those of the other Thames River company such that each supplied every other house in an area of London that they both served. Snow counted the number of houses in the district served by each company and the number of cholera cases that developed in houses served by each company.

The resulting rates were greatly different, with a much higher rate of cholera in the houses served by the company that was still drawing its water from the polluted source.

This classic study reflects a design referred to as the case control method. This form of research is especially important and useful when one is trying to determine the possible cause of a disease. It has been employed widely and added to our medical knowledge in ways such as the discovery that infant deformities were in the offspring of women who had nothing in common other than ingestion of thalidomide during their pregnancy to the studies that showed a much higher incidence of lung cancer among smokers than among nonsmokers.

Much of the work that has revealed the risk factors for various cancers were obtained from case control studies that compared people with cancer to a group of people without cancer, the control group, which was matched in age, sex, and so on with the disease or case group. Middle-aged women in Aurora, Illinois, were reported to have bone cancer more than women in surrounding communities. They seemed like the other women except that they had all worked at a radium dial watch factory in Aurora some years previously, whereas none of the cancer-free control group had worked with the radium. The conclusion was that exposure to radioactive material is a risk factor for developing bone cancer.

Because of modern developments in statistical analysis, researchers also determine possible risk factors when more than one is operative. Such analysis would be used with large cross-sectional community studies that record the prevalence of a disease and other characteristics of the population. The Framingham heart study was of this sort. It revealed that people with heart disease tend to have hypertension, elevated cholesterol readings, and a history of smoking more than those who do not suffer from heart disease.

A follow-up study conducted for several years is currently recording the practices of the offspring of the original study population and the development of heart disease among them. This type of study is called a cohort incidence study because it looks for the development of disease over time. Expensive and lengthy, it is also sometimes impractical.

Each of these designs is useful when one is trying to find the cause of a disease, especially a disease that develops slowly over time. Another type of design that is useful to determine the best form of treatment for a disease is the clinical trial. Some professionals erroneously regard this design as more scientific than the others because the investigator has some control over the exposure of the test sample to a given factor, a treatment of some sort, but this view is incorrect. The randomized controlled trial is subject to many of the same biases as the other designs that I discuss in my article, "The case control or retrospective study in retrospect," *Journal of Clinical Pharmacology* 21:269–274, July 1981. The debate is moot, however, because the clinical trial cannot be used to determine the cause of a disease. No one can ethically subject healthy people to a factor suspected of causing a disease.

An early example of a clinical trial that *did* test various treatments and also determined the cause of a disease was an investigation made by James Lind into the treatment of scurvy among English sailors in 1747. Sailors long away at sea were afflicted with debilitating scurvy because fresh fruits and vegetables were not storable aboard ship for long periods, and they lacked vitamin C when they went on long voyages.

Lind, on board the *Salisbury*, gathered sailors who were suffering from scurvy and divided them into several groups matched for severity and other factors. He then required that one group take 25 gutts of elixir vitriol daily, another group 2 spoonfuls of vinegar three times daily, another nutmeg, another oranges and lemons, while another group was allowed only a ration of seawater. Within days, dramatic change for the better occurred only in those eating the oranges and lemons.

Lind concluded that eating citrus fruits was essential to the diet of anyone who wished to avoid scurvy and that the disease was caused by the lack of these same fruits in the diet. The British Navy adopted the policy of serving its sailors limes and lime juice in 1795.

This experiment led Lind to the cause as well as to the treatment of scurvy, yet he did not choose to cause scurvy in the sailors by withholding citrus fruits from the sailors. They were already sick. In this instance, he felt no compunction about giving one group only seawater, which he regarded tantamount to no treatment, a strategy employed today usually with a group of sick people that constitutes a control group.

Ethical considerations can affect such decisions, and often such experiments avoid having a no-treatment group in favor of having several groups each treated differently but all treated with some accepted treatment. The groups are called comparison groups and provide data on which treatment of several possible ones is the best.

The data in *Cancer* present survival information collected from clinical treatment trials as researchers search for the most effective way to fight this disease. Some patients are given chemotherapy in different ways, some radiation treatments in different doses, others undergo surgery, and some receive all three when there is indication that these modalities in combination offer some success. As noted, survival for victims of a given kind of cancer can vary considerably, depending on the treatment.

Readers mindful of these many considerations and of the strategies used by medical researchers to determine what disease patterns exist and how they reveal possible causes of disease will better evaluate the information in this series. They will also better understand why controversy often rages within the medical community about the causes or treatment of disease. And they will better appreciate the remarkable progress achieved by epidemiologists, medical researchers, treating physicians, and policy makers in increasing average life expectancy and eliminating much pain and suffering from normal human existence.

Glossary

Addition: the readmission to inpatient care after release from treatment initiated during the same year; the return from short term leave; or the transfer from outpatient or day treatment to inpatient care; an outpatient or day treatment addition is each admission or readmission to the same care setting or a transfer from another type of care setting

Age-adjusted rate: age adjustment, using the direct method, is the application of the age-specific death rates in a population of interest to a standardized age distribution to eliminate the differences in observed rates that result from differences in population composition

Average daily census: the ratio of the total annual inpatient days, excluding passes and leaves, divided by 365

Average length of stay: the patient days not counting the day of discharge per patient discharged during a given period

Beds: inpatient beds set up and staffed for use at the end of a calendar year

Catatonic: stuporous, rigid form of schizophrenia

Cohort: any group of people with a common characteristic or set of characteristics studied or followed over time

Death rate: a measure that divides the number of deaths in a population in a given period by the resident population at the middle of that period

Discharge: release from care or transfer to a non-inpatient department or nonpsychiatric ward of non-federal general hospital but not death

Dysthymia: melancholia; dysfunction of the thyroid gland

First listed diagnosis: the first diagnosis on a hospital discharge summary or other document; the primary diagnosis

Full-time staff: non-trainees working 35 or more hours weekly

Incidence: the number of cases of disease having their onset during a particular interval, often expressed as a rate

Length of stay: the days between admission and discharge with those admitted and discharged on the same day counted as a 1-day stay

Life expectancy: the average years of life remaining to a person at a particular age based generally on the mortality conditions existing in the time mentioned

Lifetime prevalence: the proportion of persons in a representative sample of the population who have *ever* experienced that disorder up to the date of assessment

Marital status: unmarried typically includes those who are single (never married), divorced, or widowed, but the abortion surveillance reports of the Atlanta Centers for Disease Control count separated people as unmarried for all states except Rhode Island

Noninstitutionalized population: the population not residing in correctional institutions, detention homes, and training schools for delinquents, homes for the aged and dependent, homes for neglected children, the mentally or physically handicapped, unwed mothers, psychiatric or tuberculosis, and chronic disease hospitals. This population is the denominator in rates calculated for the National Center for Health Statistics' National Health Interview Survey, National Health and Nutrition Examination Survey, and National Ambulatory Medical Care Survey.

Pathology: study of the nature and cause of disease

Patient-care episodes: patients under care plus additions in a given year

Prevalence: the cases of a disease, number of infected persons, or persons with some other attribute present during a particular interval; often expressed as a rate

Resident population: the population living in the United States including armed forces and resident foreigners excluding diplomats

Schizophreniform: a disorder similar to schizophrenia, lasting 1

to 6 weeks and classified separately because of its better prognosis

Six-month prevalence: disturbance that the DIS indicates as active in the six months prior to interview

Somatization: a type of bodily disorder arising from a deep-seated neurotic cause similar to conversion

Bibliography

AMA: *The Recognition of Jail Inmates with Mental Illness, Their Special Problems and Needs for Care.* 1977 (hereafter *AMA, Recognition*)

American Psychiatric Association Task Force on Drug Dependence. Position statement on guidelines for methadone maintenance treatment by private psychiatrists. *Psychiat* 128: 254–255, 1971

Aronow R, Done AK: Phencyclidine overdose: an emerging concept of management. *JACEP* 7: 56–59, 1978

Block GD, Page TL: Circadian pacemakers in the nervous system. *Ann Rev Neuroscience* 1:19–34, 1978

Bunney WE, Jr. (moderator):   The switch process in manic-depressive psychosis. *Ann Intern Med* 87:319–335, 1977

Caparulo Barbara K, Cohen DJ: Cognitive structures, language, and emerging social competence in autistic and aphasic children. *Child Psychiat* 1977, in press

Celani D: An interpersonal approach to hysteria. *Am J Psychiat* 133(12):1414–1418, 1976

Chesser ES: Behaviour therapy: recent trends and current practice. *Br J Psychiat*, 129:289–307, 1976

Cohen DJ: *Childhood Autism and Atypical Development.* Taboroff Memorial Lecture, University of Utah School of Medicine,

1975

Cohen DJ, Caparulo BK, Shaywitz, BA: *Neurochemical and Developmental Models of Childhood Autism.* Presented at meeting of Kittay Scientific Foundation, New York, April 1977, in press

Cohen DJ, Caparulo K, Shaywitz, BA: Primary childhood aphasia and childhood autism: clinical, biological, and conceptual observations. *J Am Acad Child Psychiat* 15(4): 604–645, 1976

Cohen DJ, Young JG: Neurochemistry and child psychiatry. *J Am Child Psychiat* 16(3): 353–411, 1977

Cohen DJ: The diagnostic process in child psychiatry. *Psychiatri Ann* 6(9):September 1976

Cohen S, Gallant DM: *Diagnosis of Drug and Alcohol Abuse* (National Training System Medical Monograph Vol. 1, No. 6). Manuscript submitted for publication, 1981

Colman JC: *Abnormal Psychology and Modern Life*, 4th ed. Glenview, Ill.: Scott, Foresman, 1972

Cox D: *Modern Psychology: The Teachings of Carl Gustav Jung.* New York: Barnes & Noble, 1968

Crosby JF: Theories of anxiety: a theoretical perspective. *Am J Psychoanal* 36(3):237–248, 1976

Davis J, Sekerke J, Janowski D: Drug interactions involving drugs of abuse. In National Commission on Marijuana and Drug Use, *Drug Use in America: Problem in Perspective* (Second report of the National Commission on Marijuana and Drug Use). Washington, D.C.: U.S. Government Printing Office, 1973

Dole VP, Nyswander M: A medical treatment for diacetylmorphine (heroin) addiction: a clinical trial with methadone hydrochloride. *JAMA*, 193, 646–650, 1965

Dyrud J: Toward a science of the passions. *Saturday Rev* 22–27, February 21, 1976

Eysenck HJ: *The Dynamics of Anxiety and Hysteria: An Experimental Application of Modern Learning Theory to Psychiatry.* New York: Praeger, 1957

Feldman LB: Depression and marital interaction. *Family Process* 15(4): 389–395,1976

Fultz JM, Senay EC: Guidelines for the management of hospitalized narcotic addicts. *Ann Intern Med* 82: 815–818, 1975

Galton L: How to overcome a phobia. *Parade,* August 8, 1976

Gay GR, Senay EC, Newmeyer JA: The pseudo junkie: evolution of heroin life-style in the non-addicted individual. *Drug Forum* 2:279–290, 1973

Gold PW, Goodwin FK, Reus V: Vasopressin in affective illness. *Lancet* 1:1233–1236, 1978

Goldstein A, Judson BA: Efficacy and side effects of three widely different methadone doses. In *Proceedings of the Fifth National Conference on Methadone Treatment.* New York: National Association for the Prevention of Addiction to Narcotics, 1973

Goodwin FK: Diagnosis of affective disorders. In Jarvik, ME (ed.): *Psychopharmacology in the Practice of Medicine.* New York: Appleton-Century-Crofts, pp. 219–227, 1977

Goodwin FK, Post RM: Studies of amine metabolites in affective illness and in schizophrenia: A comparative analysis. In Freedman D (ed.): *The Biology of the Major Psychoses.* New York: Raven Press, pp. 299–332, 1975

Gorlow L, Katkovsky W (eds.) *Readings in the Psychology of Adjustment,* 2d ed. New York: McGraw-Hill, 1968

Gratz RR: Accidental injury in childhood: a literature review on pediatric trauma. *J Trauma* 19: 551–555, August 1979

Griffin JB: The psychiatric examination. In Walker HK, Hall WD, Hurst JW (eds.) *Clinical Methods: The History, Physical, and Laboratory Examinations.* Boston: Butterworths, 1976

Grof P, Angst J, Haines T: The clinical course of practical issues. *Symposia Medica Hoechst 8: Classification and Prediction of Outcome of Depression.* New York: Schattauer Verlag, pp. 141–148 1974

Grof P; Zis AP, Goodwin FK et al: *Patterns of Recurrence in Bipolar Affective Illness.* Paper presented at the Annual Meeting of the American Psychiatric Association, Atlanta, Georgia, May 1978

Guillemin R: New endocrinology of the brain. *Perspect Bio Med*, Part 2, 22 (2):S74–S80, 1979

Jaffe JH, Zaks MS, Washington EN: Experience with the use of methadone in a multi-modality program for the treatment of narcotics users. *Internat J Addictions*, 4:481–490, 1969

Johnson MS: Effect of continuous light on periodic spontaneous activity of white-footed mice. *J Exp Zool* 82:315, 1939

Johnson RE: *Existential Man: The Challenge of Psychotherapy.* Elmsford, N.Y.: Pergamon Press, 1971

Jung CG: *Modern Man in Search of a Soul.* (1911) Translated by W.S. Dell and Cary F. Baynes. New York: Harcourt, Brace and World

Kanfer FH, Karoly P: Self-control: a behavioristic excursion into the lion's den. *Behav Ther* 3(3): 398–416,1972

Kassirer JP: Serious acid-base disorders. *N Engl J Med* 291:773–776, 1974

Klemesrud J: Conquering a phobia that makes a healthy woman stay home. *The New York Times*, August 6, 1976

Kline NS: *From Sad to Glad.* New York: G.P. Putnam's Sons, 1974

Kotulak R: Too much of a bad thing may cure that neurosis. *Chicago Tribune*, June 27, 1976

Kotulak R: Your defenses: ego trip up or down. *Chicago Tribune*, August 1, 1976

Kraepelin E: *Manic-Depressive Insanity and Paranoia.* Translated by M. Barklay, edited by G.M. Robertson. Edinburgh: E. and S. Livingston, 1921

Lewy AJ, Wehr T, Goodwin F: Plasma melatonin in manic-depressive illness. *NIMH Abstract,* 1979

Lindzey G, Hall CS (eds.): *Theories of Personality: Primary Sources and Research.* New York: John Wiley & Sons, 1965

Loew CA, Grayson H; Loew GH: *Three Psychotherapies: A Clinical Comparison.* New York: Brunner/Mazel, 1975

London P: The end of ideology in behavior modification. *Am Psychol* 27(10): 913–920, 1972

Malin HJ, Munch NE: *Implicated Alcohol and Disease Entities, Alcohol as a Risk Factor in the Nation's Health.* Report of the Alcohol Epidemiologic Data System. Contract No. ADM 281-79-0012. Prepared for the National Institute on Alcohol Abuse and Alcoholism, Alcohol, Drug Abuse, and Mental Health Administration. Rockville, Md., March 28, 1980

Martin B: *Anxiety and Neurotic Disorders.* New York: John Wiley & Sons, 1971

Maslow AH: *The Farther Reaches of Human Nature.* New York: Viking Press, 1971

McMahon FB: *Abnormal Behavior: Psychology's View.* Englewood Cliffs, N.J.: Prentice-Hall, 1976

McNeil EB: *Neuroses and Personality Disorders.* Englewood Cliffs, N.J.: Prentice-Hall, 1970

Mehndiratta SS, Wig NN: Psychosocial effects of long term cannabis use in India. *Drug and Alcohol Dependence* 1:71–82, 1975

Mozdzierz GJ, Macchitelli FJ, Lisiecki J: The paradox in psychotherapy: an Adlerian perspective. *J Individ Psych* 32(2): 169–185, 1976

Myers JK, Weissman MM, Tischler GL et al: Six-month prevalence of psychiatric disorders in three communities, *Archives of General Psychiatry,* Vol. 41, No. 10, Oct. 1984

National Institute on Alcohol Abuse and Alcoholism: alcohol use and alcohol problems among U.S. adults. Results of the 1979 national survey, by W. B. Clark and L. Midanik. *Alcohol and Health Monograph No. 1, Alcohol Consumption and Related Problems.*

DHHS Pub. No. (ADM) 82-1190. Alcohol, Drug Abuse, and Mental Health Administration. Washington. U.S. Government Printing Office, 1982a.

National Institute on Alcohol Abuse: *Student Drug Abuse in America 1975-1982.* DHHS Pub. No. (ADM) 83-1260. Rockville, MD. NIDA, 1983b.

O'Brien JS, Raynes AE, Patch VD: Treatment of heroin addiction with aversion therapy, relaxation training and systematic desensitization. *Behav Res Ther* 10: 77–80, 1972

O'Donnell JA: *Narcotic addicts in Kentucky.* (U.S. Public Health Service Publication No. 1881.) Washington, D.C.: U.S. Government Printing Office, 1969

Piaget J, Inhelder B: *The Psychology of the Child.* Translated by Helen Weaver. New York: Basic Books, 1969

Rachman S: *Phobias, Their Nature and Control.* Springfield, Ill.: CC Thomas, 1968

Rachman S: The modification of obsessions: a new formulation: *Behav Res Ther* 14(6): 437–445, 1976

Rachman S, Roper G: The spontaneous decay of compulsive urges. *Behav Res Ther* 14(6): 445–455, 1976

Raynes AE, Patch VD, Cohen M: Comparison of opiate and polydrug abusers in treatment. *J Psychedel Drugs* 7:135–141, 1975

Robins JS,   Helzer JE et al: Lifetime prevalence of specific psychiatric disorders in three sites, *Archives of General Psychiatry*, Vol. 41 No. 10, Oct. 1984

Robins LN: Etiological implications in studies of childhood histories relating to antisocial personality. In Hare RD, Schalling D (eds.): *Psychopathic Behavior.* New York: Wiley, in press

Robins LN: Antisocial behavior disturbances of childhood: prevalence, prognosis, and prospects. In Koupernik A (ed.): *The Child in His Family—Children at a Psychiatric Risk.* New York: Wiley, 1974

Robins LN: *Deviant Children Grown Up.* Baltimore: Williams and Wilkins, 1966. Reprinted by Robert E. Krieger Publishing Co., Huntington, N.Y., 1974

Robins LN: Follow-up studies investigating childhood disorders. In Hare EH, Wing JK (eds.): *Psychiatric Epidemiology.* London: Oxford University Press, 1970

Robins, LN, Lewis RG: The role of the antisocial family in school completion and delinquency: a three-generation study. *Sociol Q* 7:500–514, 1966

Robins LN, West PA, Herjanic BL: Arrests and delinquency in two generations: a study of black urban families and their children. *J Child Psychol Psychiat* 16: 125–140, 1975

Robins LN, Wish E: Childhood deviance as a developmental process: a study of 223 urban black men from birth to 18. *Social Forces*, December 1977

Rosen E, Gregory I: *Abnormal Psychology.* Philadelphia: W.B. Saunders, 1965

Rosenfeld A: And now, preventive psychiatry. *Sat Rev* 24–25, February 21, 1976

Rothgeb CL (ed.): *Abstracts of the Standard Edition of the Complete Psychological Works of Sigmund Freud.* DHEW Pub. No. (HSM) 72-9001. Washington, D.C.: Superintendent of Documents, U.S. Government Printing Office, 1972

Rubin V, Comitas L: *Ganja in Jamaica.* Paris: Mouton, 1975

Rusak B, Zucker I: Biological rhythms and animal behavior. *Ann Rev Psycho* 26:137–171, 1975

Rutter M: Parent-child separation: psychological effects on the children. *J Child Psychiat* 12:233–260, 1971

Ryle A: *Neurosis in the Ordinary Family.* London: Tavistock, 1967

Salzman L: *The Obsessive Personality: Origins, Dynamics, and Therapy.* New York: Science House, 1968

Skinner BF: *About Behaviorism,* New York: Knopf, 1974

Smith, D.E: *Polydrug Abuse and Comprehensive Treatment Intervention.* Rockville, Maryland: National Clearinghouse for Drug Abuse Information, 1976

Snyder, S. *Madness and the Brain.* New York: McGraw-Hill, 1974

Snyder S: *The Troubled Mind: A Guide to Release from Distress.* New York: McGraw-Hill, 1976

Suinn RM: *Fundamentals of Behavior Pathology,* (2d ed). New York: Wiley, 1975

Taub JM, Berger RJ: Acute shifts in the sleep-wakefulness cycle: Effects on performance and mood. *Psycho Med* 36:164–173, 1974

Tennant FS, Jr: Drug abuse in the US Army, Europe. *JAM,* 221:1146–1149, 1972

Tennant FS, Jr: Propoxyphene napsylate (Darvon-N) treatment of heroin addicts. *J National Med Assoc* 66:23–24, 27, 1974

Thorne FC: A new approach to psychopathology. *J Clin Psycholo* 32(4): 751–756, 1976

Turner, LB (ed): *National Conference of Commissioners on Uniform State Laws: Handbook and Proceedings.* Chicago: National Conference on Commissioners on Uniform State Laws, 1973

Ullman LP, Krasner L: *A Psychological Approach to Abnormal Behavior,* (2d ed). Englewood Cliffs: Prentice-Hall, 1975

Vaillant GE: A 20-year follow-up study of New York narcotic addicts. *Arc Gen Psychiat* 29:237–241, 1973

Vaillant GE: Natural history of male psychological health. V. The relationship of choice of ego mechanisms of defense to adult adjustment. *Arch Gen Psychiat* 33:535–545, 1976

Wallace RK: Physiological effects of transcendental meditation. *Science* 167: 1751–1754, 1970

Wehr, TA: Phase and biorhythm studies of affective illness. In Bunney W (moderator): The Switch Process in Manic-Depressive Psychosis. *Ann Intern Med* 87:321–324, 1977

Wehr, TA, Goodwin FK: Catecholamines in depression. In Burrows GD (ed.): *Handbook of Studies in Depression.* New York: Elsevier-North Holland, 1977

Wehr, TA, Goodwin FK: Rapid cycling in manic depressives induced by tricyclic antidepressants. *Arch Gen Psychiatr* 36:555–559, 1979

Wehr, TA, Goodwin FK: Biological rhythms and affective illness. *Weekly Psychiatry Update Series* 2:(28)2–7, 1978

Weitzman ED, Czeisler CA, Moore-Ede M: Sleep-wake neuroendocrine and body temperature circadian rhythms under entrained and non-entrained free-running conditions in man. NATO International Symposium on Biorhythms and Its Central Mechanism, Tokyo. New York: Elsevier-North Holland, in press

Weitzman ED, Nogeire C, Perlow M et al: Effects of a prolonged 3-hour sleep-wake cycle on sleep stage, plasma cortisol, growth hormone and body temperature in man. *J Clini Endocrinol Metab* 38:1018–1070, 1974

Wever R: *The Circadian System in Man.* New York: Springer Verlag, 1979

Wieland WF, Novack JL: A comparison of criminal justice and noncriminal justice related patients in a methadone treatment program. In *Proceedings of the Fifth National Conference on Methadone Treatment.* New York: National Association for the Prevention of Addiction to Narcotics, 1973

Wolpe J: *The Practice of Behavior Therapy.* New York: Pergamon Press, 1969

Woodruff RA, Goodwin DW, Guze SB: *Psychiatric Diagnosis.* New York: Oxford University Press, 1974

Wurtman RJ, Moskowitz MA: The pineal organ, (two parts). *New Eng J Med* 296:1329–1333, 1383–1386, 1977

Zis AP, Goodwin FK: Major affective disorder as a recurrent illness. *Arch Gen Psychiat* 36:835–839, 1979

Zis A, Groff P, Webster M et al: Prediction of relapse in recurrent affective disorder. *Psychopharmaco Bull* 16 (1), 1980

INDEX